Pivotal Response Treatment for Autism

A Guide for Support Providers

Pivotal Response Treatment for Autism

A Guide for Support Providers

Lynn Kern Koegel, Ph.D.

Clinical Professor, Department of Psychiatry and Behavioral Sciences, Stanford University School of Medicine, Stanford, California; Editor, *Journal of Autism and Developmental Disorders*

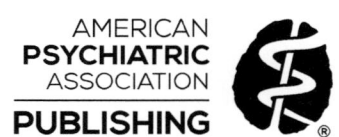

AMERICAN
PSYCHIATRIC
ASSOCIATION
PUBLISHING

Copyright © 2025 American Psychiatric Association Publishing

ALL RIGHTS RESERVED

First Edition

Manufactured in the United States of America on acid-free paper
29 28 27 26 25   5 4 3 2 1
American Psychiatric Association Publishing
800 Maine Avenue SW, Suite 900
Washington, DC 20024–2812
www.appi.org

Library of Congress Cataloging-in-Publication Data
Names: Koegel, Lynn Kern, author. | American Psychiatric Association Publishing, publisher.
    Title: Pivotal response treatment for autism : a guide for support providers / Lynn Kern Koegel.
Description: First edition. | Washington, DC : American Psychiatric Association Publishing, [2025] | Includes bibliographical references and index.
Identifiers: LCCN 2024059461 (print) | LCCN 2024059462 (ebook) | ISBN 9798894550879 (paperback ; alk. paper) | ISBN 9798894550886 (ebook) | ISBN 9798894550893 (epub)
Subjects: MESH: Autistic Disorder--therapy | Language Therapy | Communication | Case Reports
Classification: LCC RC553.A88 (print) | LCC RC553.A88 (ebook) | NLM WS 350.8.P4 | DDC 616.85/882--dc23/eng/20250307
LC record available at https://lccn.loc.gov/2024059461
LC ebook record available at https://lccn.loc.gov/2024059462

British Library Cataloguing in Publication Data

A CIP record is available from the British Library.

Contents

Preface

Pivotal response treatment (PRT) is an evidence-based intervention for autism spectrum disorder (ASD). Publications discussing this intervention package began appearing in the 1980s, and hundreds of articles from centers around the world support this intervention for various behaviors that interfere with the development of communication, learning, and socialization. PRT was developed in response to the commonly used applied behavior analysis (ABA) interventions that incorporated repetitive, drill-type practice, such that the children became unmotivated to respond and engaged in high levels of interfering avoidance and escape behavior. We found that when we incorporated specific motivational components into the intervention, greater gains were achieved and concomitant changes in untargeted areas were seen, which resulted in better outcomes. Motivation was the first area researched, and our team found that when specific motivational components were incorporated into the intervention, children on the autism spectrum responded better and with more correct responses.

Initially, our work on motivation was focused on improving the communication of largely nonverbal children with ASD and was named the *natural language paradigm* because it closely resembled the way neurotypical children learn language. However, once the research showed that motivational procedures could be applied to areas other than communication, it was renamed *pivotal response treatment*. Pivotal areas are those that, once taught, result in positive improvements in other areas that are not specifically targeted. These keystone areas are critical to accelerating learning and improving engagement. Since the initial discovery of the pivotal area of motivation, other pivotal areas have been discovered, including initiations, self-management, and, more recently, empathetic responding.

Regarding terminology, opinions vary regarding whether person-first (e.g., *child with autism*) or identity-first (e.g., *autistic adult*) language should be used. When I first started working in the field, we exclusively used identity-first language (e.g., *autistic child*). However, in the late 1970s and early 1980s, parents expressed a strong desire for person-first language. A quick search of the literature shows how the terminology changed over that decade in response to these parents' wishes (Zajic and Gudknecht 2024). More recently, highly verbal individuals who view autism as part of their identity have preferred identity-first language (*autistic person*); however, people who have experienced stigma related to their autism find identity-first language less preferable or offensive (Bury et al. 2023). Culture may influence this preference as well; research shows that individuals and parents in countries other than the United States often prefer person-first language (e.g., Buijsman et al. 2023). In my own research, I ask participants or their families what they would like me to use. Most of the adolescents and adults I have asked do not have a strong preference, but families of young children often prefer person-first language. Therefore, out of respect for the diversity of opinions, I have used both approaches to terminology in this book.

I hope you find this book helpful in your work. We continue on a research mission to improve services with the hope of enhancing outcomes for individuals on the autism spectrum. As we move toward more person-/child-centered interventions—a trend that gained momentum in the 1980s so that the learning process would be more meaningful and enjoyable—we find that these procedures are also more acceptable to autistic individuals. As you read this book, please use your creativity to guide interventions toward incorporating the PRT motivational components into target behaviors so that gains are more rapid and so that children and families can enjoy the process.

References

Buijsman R, Begeer S, Scheeren AM: "Autistic person" or "person with autism"? Person-first language preference in Dutch adults with autism and parents. Autism 27(3):788–795, 2023 35957517

Bury SM, Jellett R, Haschek A, et al: Understanding language preference: autism knowledge, experience of stigma and autism identity. Autism 27(6):1588–1600, 2023 36510834

Zajic MC, Gudknecht J: Person- and identity-first language in autism research: a systematic analysis of abstracts from 11 autism journals. Autism 28(10):2445–2461, 2024 38570904

1

Autism Overview and the Development of Pivotal Response Treatment

Autism: The Label

Autism was first recognized as a distinct category in 1943, when Austrian-born child psychiatrist Leo Kanner described 11 children (8 boys and 3 girls) who were being seen in his practice at Johns Hopkins Hospital and who presented in a manner uniquely different from patients with any other condition previously reported. His journal publication describing these children was titled "Autistic Disturbances in Affective Contact" (Kanner 1943), and although the children's individual characteristics varied, he described them all as having the "inability" to relate to other people and situations, starting from "the

1

beginning of life." He also reported that the parents described their children as "happiest when left alone," "self-sufficient," "in a shell," and "failing to develop the usual amount of social awareness." He noted that some were delayed in learning to speak, and 3 of the 11 were reported to be nonverbal. Those who did learn verbal communication were reportedly unable to use that communication to convey meaning to others. He noted that no specific physical features distinguished the children, and most of the children who were verbal used clear articulation. In this publication, Kanner also remarked that the parents of these children were not warmhearted, and he questioned whether this may have led to their condition. This prompted interest in the parental causation theory, which subsequently led to autism being considered and categorized as a form of childhood schizophrenia presumably caused by the parents.

During the 1950s and 1960s, the sentiment that this condition resulted from cold, unemotional mothers who (either consciously or unconsciously) did not want their child to live persisted, particularly following publications by another Austrian-born American psychologist, Bruno Bettelheim (1967). Bettelheim's theories were partly based on his experience in concentration camps during World War II. He described the relationships between the Nazi guards and prisoners as being similar to the experiences of a child with autism—that is, like the guards, these children's mothers had toxic relationships with them and did not provide them with emotional support. This caused the children to isolate themselves and withdraw, resulting in an "empty fortress." Bettelheim theorized that this lack of early parental support made children on the autism spectrum unable to become independent. Although some blame also was placed on the fathers, the mothers took the larger brunt and were dubbed "refrigerator mothers." Consequently, most children with this condition were separated from their mothers, and this removal was termed a "parentectomy." Bettelheim argued that the early psychological damage created by these negative parental interactions during the critical early stages of development had to be reversed. His "milieu therapy" involved admitting patients into a nonthreatening residential treatment environment where they could feel comfortable expressing themselves and, in turn, socializing with others.

Clearly, many objective explanations have debunked this early parental causation theory. Personality tests of parents of children with autism show that they are no different from parents of neurotypical children, a fact that has been demonstrated repeatedly over many decades (R.L. Koegel et al. 1983). However, parents may experience stress and other issues related to the challenges of having a child on the spectrum (Gau et al. 2012). Additionally, evidence indicating that genetic or chromosomal abnormalities are a cause of autism includes autism being four times more likely to be diagnosed in males[1] (Loomes et al. 2017); identical twins almost always both presenting with autism (Bohm et al. 2013); and rates of autism or similar conditions being shown to be higher within families (Vashisth and Chahrour 2023). A variety of other potential environmental risk factors also may play a role in the development of autism, although the cause or causes and mechanisms have not yet been elucidated (Lu et al. 2022). Overall, the wide variety of characteristics in individuals diagnosed with autism, especially in large group studies where characteristics may not be specifically defined, makes this research challenging.

Although theories of the root cause of autism have changed dramatically, the characteristics of autism spectrum disorder (ASD) as described by Kanner (1943) have largely remained the same. The three major domains he described—qualitative impairments in reciprocal social interaction, impairments in communication, and restricted interests that include resistance to change and repetitive movements—continue to define the condition today. According to DSM-5 (American Psychiatric Association 2013, 2022), individuals diagnosed with ASD show 1) persistent differences in social communication and social interaction and 2) restricted and repetitive patterns of behavior, interests, or activities. These behaviors must be present early on (even if they fully manifest later when social demands increase), must significantly interfere with daily living, and must not be better explained by an intellectual disability or global developmental delay (although other conditions frequently co-occur with ASD). Although other behaviors, such as meltdowns and aggression, may develop or continue from early childhood, they are not part of the diagnostic criteria. Similarly, eating and sleeping disorders are common in individuals with autism but are not part of the diagnostic criteria.

The diagnosis of Asperger's disorder also has come and gone over the decades. The year after Kanner (1943) published his paper using the term *autism*, Hans Asperger (1944) published a paper entitled "Autistic Psychopathy in Childhood," written in German, wherein he described four boys with common characteristics that also appeared to differ

---

[1] Some have suggested that this rate may be closer to three times more likely due to gender bias (Cruz et al. 2024).

from those of other conditions. This article received little attention until the 1980s, when Lorna Wing, a British autism researcher, began to discuss this as a subtype of autistic individuals. She later translated Asperger's article into English (Wing 1981, 1991). Patients with this subtype were described as being highly intelligent but limited by difficulty with social interaction, a lack of affection, challenges with socialization, and narrow interests. Behavioral concerns, prosody issues, and hypersensitivities to sound, taste, and textures also may be present in some patients. However, Kanner (1943) remarked that this phenotype was not unique and that many autistic individuals who were intellectually "intact" excelled in professions related to their interests. Asperger also discussed the difficulty in testing these children because of their "uneven knowledge" and described them as having "autistic intelligence." Unlike Kanner and Bettelheim, Asperger suggested that autism may be a hereditary condition. Awareness of this subgroup led to the subcategory of Asperger's disorder being added to DSM-IV (American Psychiatric Association 1994), although it waslater removed from DSM-5.

Historical Events Relating to the Autism Diagnosis

Regarding the history of the diagnosis, autism was not listed in DSM as a distinct category until DSM-III (American Psychiatric Association 1980). Prior to that, it was considered a form of childhood schizophrenia. Thus, although it did exist in case reports, it did not appear in its own category of diagnosis. Table 1.1 provides a brief timeline of the iterations of the autism diagnosis. The section that follows ("The DSM Criteria") discusses the current diagnostic criteria for ASD.

The DSM Criteria

Currently, DSM-5 lists the diagnostic characteristics described for ASD. The italicized criteria that follow are taken directly from DSM-5. Although many of the criteria overlap to some extent, case examples have been provided to describe various expressions of the characteristics and to emphasize the heterogeneity of the spectrum.

Table 1.1 History of events related to autism diagnosis

1943	Leo Kanner, M.D., publishes "Autistic Disturbances in Affective Contact" in the journal *Nervous Child*, describing 11 children with various cognitive, social, linguistic, and behavioral characteristics that were different from any previously described condition.
1944	Hans Asperger, M.D., publishes an article entitled "Autistic Psychopathy in Childhood" in a German journal, *Archiv für Psychiatrie und Nervenkrankheiten*, that describes four children who had significant challenges with socialization (primary challenge), imagination, and communication (although first words may be evidenced at expected ages) and poor motor coordination but demonstrated outstanding intelligence in specific areas.
1950	Bruno Bettelheim, Ph.D., writes *Love is Not Enough: The Treatment of Emotionally Disturbed Children*. In this book, he suggests that challenging behaviors are a consequence of the child's environment, that many emotional problems are caused by the parents, and that "emotionally disturbed" children must be separated and protected from their parents. His therapy was designed for children who did not have a "normal attachment or relationship," particularly with their mothers.
1964	Bernard Rimland, Ph.D., parent of an autistic son, writes *Infantile Autism: The Syndrome and Its Implications for a Neural Theory of Behavior*, in which he criticizes the parental causation theory alluded to in previous publications and describes autism as a biological disorder.
1967	Bruno Bettelheim publishes *The Empty Fortress: Infantile Autism and the Birth of the Self*, in which he suggests that childhood frustrations caused by parents (particularly mothers) during the oral and anal phases of the child's development lead to a vicious circle of the parent(s) not wanting the child and the child sensing parental rejection, ultimately resulting in autism. This once-popular book discusses psychogenic theory in relation to autism and results in the widespread adoption of this notion.
1968	DSM-II (American Psychiatric Association 1968) adds the diagnosis of schizophrenia, childhood type, for which the diagnostic criteria include "autistic, atypical and withdrawn behavior, failure to develop identity separate from the mother, and general unevenness, gross immaturity and inadequacy in development, with an onset before puberty." Thereafter, most autistic children are diagnosed under this category.

Table 1.1 History of events related to autism diagnosis *(continued)*

1980	Infantile autism is first listed in DSM-III as its own category under the pervasive developmental disorders (PDDs). No longer is the condition associated with schizophrenia. Characteristics include 1) qualitative impairments in reciprocal social interaction, 2) impairments in communication, and 3) restricted interests, resistance to change, and repetitive movements, all developing before the age of 30 months.
1981	Lorna Wing, M.D., translates Hans Asperger's 1944 German paper into English. Following this publication, the distinction between autism and Asperger's disorder gains momentum and becomes widely accepted.
1987	DSM-III is revised and published as DSM-III-R (American Psychiatric Association 1987). The category of autism is greatly expanded to include various levels of the diagnostic characteristics, particularly on the mild end (describing it as PDD). The age at onset criterion (before 30 months) is dropped. Although the term *spectrum* is not used, the category suggests a wider variety of characteristics.
1994	DSM-IV is published, and autism is categorized as a spectrum. Autistic disorder is placed under the general category of PDD (which is not a diagnostic category but an umbrella term), along with PDD not otherwise specified. The additional categories of Asperger's disorder, child disintegrative disorder, and Rett syndrome are added, thus establishing five separate categories of autism.
2013	DSM-5 eliminates a number of categories and includes only autism spectrum disorder. It also combines the social and communication criteria, narrowing the three diagnostic criteria to two.

The first three criteria are part of Criterion A in DSM and relate to challenges with social communication. Each of these three criteria must be observed, either currently or by history, across multiple contexts.

1. Deficits in social-emotional reciprocity, ranging, for example, from abnormal social approach and failure of normal back-and-forth conversation; to reduced sharing of interests, emotions, or affect; to failure to initiate or respond to social interactions.

Case Example: Evan

Evan's family lived in Los Angeles. He was a quiet infant and, because of his calm temperament and tranquil demeanor, his parents hired a talent agent who secured many jobs for him in movies and television shows. However, shortly before his first birthday they noticed that he paid little attention to others, smiled infrequently, and did not respond to his name being called. He did not appear to enjoy common parent-child activities, such as "peek-a-boo" and "pat-a-cake." Although he sat up at 9 months and walked at 11 months, he had not begun to say any words by 18 months and rarely smiled when others attempted to play with him. Only a few toys interested him, and he did not appear to enjoy playing with them interactively, instead preferring to use them repetitively, such as turning a truck upside down and spinning the wheels or repeatedly turning the lights on and off on a light-up toy.

Case Example: Jose

According to his parents, Jose appeared to be meeting all his mile-stones during his first year of life. Although he was not a great sleeper, he sat up, walked, and laughed when tickled or thrown into the air. However, by 16 months, he did not point, did not follow a point shown by others (even when the object was nearby), and did not bring toys to his parents. Although he enjoyed toys with lights and sounds, he preferred to play with these alone and often turned his back toward his parents or any other adult who attempted to engage with him.

Case Example: Anna

Anna began to sing, count, and say her first words at expected or early time points. She enjoyed a few specific books, looking through them for lengthy periods of time; if her parents tried to engage with her while she was looking through the books, she would protest and refuse to share and would even become aggressive if they persisted. Although she verbally requested the books if they were out of her reach, she refused to engage socially once the books were in her hands. When her parents called her name, she rarely responded. Although Anna was able to use words and combine them into sentences, she primarily used that communication for protesting when others tried to engage with her and for requesting her favorite foods or items, such as her books.

2. Deficits in nonverbal communicative behaviors used for social interaction, ranging, for example, from poorly integrated verbal and nonverbal communication; to abnormalities in eye contact and body language or deficits in understanding and use of gestures; to a total lack of facial expressions and nonverbal communication.

Case Example: Rya

Since birth, Rya rarely made eye contact with others. Her parents reported that when she was an infant, she appeared to look "through them" rather than "at them." Around her first birthday, she did not respond when her parents made silly faces or actions. At age 2 years, she had not started using words or pointing but would take a parent's hand and lead them to desired items, such as by placing their hand on the doorknob when she wanted to go outside.

Case Example: Anil

Anil developed verbal communication, albeit delayed, but did not face his communicative partner when conversing and did not pick up on gestures, such as someone looking at their watch after a period of time; nor did he respond to facial expressions, such as a puzzled look or sad expression.

3. Deficits in developing, maintaining, and understanding relationships, ranging, for example, from difficulties adjusting behavior to suit various social contexts; to difficulties in sharing imaginative play or in making friends; to absence of interest in peers.

Case Example: Hao

Hao was an adolescent enrolled in mostly general education classes. He often picked his nose at school and spilled food on himself while eating. He appeared oblivious to other students nearby and often inadvertently bumped into them. He did not engage with peers without being prompted, and he paced the perimeter of the schoolyard during lunch recess. His parents reported that although he had played with the train set at preschool, he had never interacted with the other children, nor had he shared or taken turns with his toys, and playing alone had persisted into elementary school

Case Example: Jacob

> Ten-year-old Jacob reported that he had a group of friends but talked exclusively about the weather. When a peer brought up a different topic, he refused to engage, sometimes saying, "That's stupid," or "Booooooring." Although he would sit with other children and converse if they were interested in talking about the weather, he had no interest in his peers' topics of conversation.

The last four criteria are part of Criterion B and relate to restricted and repetitive patterns of behavior (RRBs), colloquially referred to as "self-stimulation" or "stim." Two of these four criteria must be observed, either currently or by history.

1. Stereotyped or repetitive motor movements, use of objects, or speech (e.g., simple motor stereotypies, lining up toys or flipping objects, echolalia, idiosyncratic phrases).

Case Example: Jenna

> Two-year-old Jenna is fascinated by lights and repetitively turns the lights of her toys on and off. Her parents report that this activity can entertain her for hours.

Case Example: Johnny

> Preschooler Johnny lines up his toys meticulously. When anyone moves a toy from the lineup, he has a meltdown. This is especially problematic when the parents have visitors with small children who play with the toys. In fact, Johnny shows visible signs of distress even when another child simply gets near his toys.

Case Example: Dominique

> Teenager Dominique's parents are both musicians, and he excels in music, but his verbal communication is limited to single words or short word combinations. He is also interested in cartoons: he repetitively watches his favorites and repeatedly recites long segments from them, such as "Bad days happen to everyone, but when one happens to you, just keep doing your best and never let a bad day make you feel bad about yourself," a passage he heard years previously on *Sesame Street*.

2. Insistence on sameness, inflexible adherence to routines, or ritualized patterns of verbal or nonverbal behavior (e.g., extreme distress at small changes, difficulties with transitions, rigid thinking patterns, greeting rituals, need to take same route or eat same food every day).

Case Example: Marisol

Preschooler Marisol comes to the clinic three times a week. The first time the family came, they entered through a side door. Because of this initial route, she insists on always entering through the same side door. If they try to enter through another door, Marisol has a meltdown until they take her around the building and enter through the side door.

Case Example: Marco

Marco engages in huge meltdowns, screaming and violently kicking the back seat of the car if his mother or father drives in any lane other than the right (slow) lane. They are unable to change lanes to pass a slow car, move to the left for an entering car, or avoid an obstacle in the road without significant behaviors. Consequently, driving with him is extremely stressful.

3. Highly restricted, fixated interests that are abnormal in intensity or focus (e.g., strong attachment to or preoccupation with unusual objects, excessively circumscribed or perseverative interests).

Case Example: Maria

Four-year-old Maria has a strong interest in numbers. She utters numbers frequently throughout the day and insists that any play activity involve numbers. For example, a toy house must have a house number in order for her to play with it. When on a walk, she calls out each house or store number and is uninterested in other topics.

Case Example: Manny

Manny carries a balloon everywhere he goes. If his parents try to encourage him to leave the balloon at home or in the car, a major meltdown follows. To avoid the meltdowns, they always carry a supply of balloons with them.

4. Hyper- or hyporeactivity to sensory input or unusual interest in sensory aspects of the environment (e.g., apparent indifference to pain/temperature, adverse response to specific sounds or textures, excessive smelling or touching of objects, visual fascination with lights or movement).

Case Example: Eric

Preschooler Eric has sound sensitivities to noises—not only loud noises but also a large variety of noises, especially toddler toys that make sounds. Unfortunately, the family cannot visit other children's homes because Eric cries hysterically even at the sight of a toy with sounds.

Case Example: Amari

Kindergartener Amari began smelling his mother's hair when he was a toddler, enjoying the scent of her shampoo. His mother did not mind this because she enjoyed the closeness when he sat on her lap, playing with her long hair and sniffing it. Now that Amari is in kindergarten, however, he repeatedly approaches the teacher, trying to sniff her hair. When she denies him, he drops to the floor and cries, sometimes for more than a half hour.

In addition to behaviorally assessing social communication and RRBs, DSM-5 recommends the evaluator note whether an intellectual disability and language delay are present (i.e., with or without intellectual impairment and language impairment).

Case Example: C.J.

C.J. began using words at an early age, and by 20 months he could recite nursery rhymes, repeat a string of numbers, and recite the alphabet. However, when he started preschool at age 2, he paid little attention to the other children, did not respond when called by his teachers, and spent a good portion of his day opening and closing the door to a small playhouse while humming. Although C.J. was precocious in his language development, his social communication was lacking.

Case Example: Melissa

Melissa sat up, crawled, and walked at an early age; however, at 2½ years of age, she was not saying any verbal expressive words, did not respond to her name being called, and had never shown any separation anxiety when her parents left her. Furthermore, she repeatedly played with a small number of toys in a nonfunctional way, turning small cars upside down and spinning the wheels or seeking out sticks, pencils, or pens to repetitively wave in front of her eyes.

Case Example: Blake

Although Blake was a late talker, he progressed nicely with his motivational language intervention program. By elementary school, his academics were on par, but his standardized test results indicated significant cognitive and language challenges. Upon closer examination, it was noted that his attention was a variable in his responsiveness. Once his attention was secured, by having him repeat instructions and giving him frequent breaks, he scored within average range on both cognitive and language tests.

Nonverbal IQ tests are often desirable for children on the autism spectrum who exhibit language challenges. In general, testing can be difficult for these children and often underestimates their functioning and potential. Some find the verbal demands frustrating but are quite adept at the nonverbal tasks. Individuals with autism range dramatically in both type and degree of their characteristics, which affects the level of support they will need in order to reach their maximum potential.

Level of Support Needed

To quantify the degree to which these characteristics impact daily activities and quality of life, DSM-5 employs a 1–3 rating scale. One score is given for social communication and another for the level to which RRBs interfere with daily living and learning.

- Level 1 indicates "requiring support," meaning that without supports in place, individuals may have difficulty initiating and responding socially and may appear to have a decreased interest in socialization. They may be able to speak in sentences and to engage communicatively, albeit with difficulty. They also may have RRBs that interfere in some contexts and may have difficulties with transitions or organization.
- Level 2 indicates "requiring substantial support," meaning that even with supports in place, these individuals may have challenges with verbal and nonverbal communication. RRBs are

obvious in various environments, and the individual exhibits some distress or difficulty when activities are changed or redirected.

- Level 3, "requiring very substantial support," is given when an individual has severe challenges in verbal and nonverbal social communication. Social responsiveness is low, and communication is significantly delayed. When scoring RRBs, the individual must demonstrate extreme discomfort or distress when activities are changed or redirected or when being asked to refocus.

These categories attempt to assess how much social communication challenges and RRBs impact an individual. They do not attempt to quantify the behaviors, such as the percentage of time RRBs are demonstrated, the percentage of time that difficulties arise when changing activities or the type of response to transitions, the number of times self-injurious or aggressive behaviors occur, or how frequently the person is unresponsive. Rather, they move toward categorizing how significantly these variables affect everyday activities.

Diagnosing a child with autism can be tricky, even at centers specializing in autism. To illustrate some of the challenges, a study of highly skilled clinicians at six highly regarded diagnostic centers in the United States (University of California San Francisco Center for Autism Spectrum and Neurodevelopmental Disorders; Seattle Children's Hospital and University of Washington; Southwest Autism Research and Resource Center; Cincinnati Children's Hospital Medical Center; Marcus Autism Center at Emory University and Children's Healthcare of Atlanta; and Rush University Medical Center) found that their diagnosticians felt some degree of uncertainty almost one-third of the time when diagnosing 16- to 30-month-old patients (Klaiman et al. 2024). Most commonly, clinicians stated that the children demonstrating only "mild" characteristics of autism made them feel most uncertain about the diagnosis. The authors of this study stated that community clinicians may experience even less certainty when diagnosing these children. This is of great importance because early intervention is critical. Such findings demonstrate the need for more precise and accurate procedures to decrease false-positive and false-negative results, which may place undue burden on families or delay treatment.

A number of autism screening measures are available, such as the Modified Checklist for Autism in Toddlers, Revised (M-CHAT-R), Childhood Autism Rating Scale (CARS), Autism Diagnostic Interview–Revised (ADI-R), and the Autism Diagnostic Observation Schedule

(ADOS), which is designed to objectively measure behavioral characteristics; however, even with these tools, clinicians report a high degree of uncertainty. More recent work suggests that artificial intelligence (AI) may be helpful in diagnosing ASD at early ages (Ghosh et al. 2021). AI studies have focused on many behavioral areas to assist with diagnosis, including (but not limited to) eye contact/tracking/gaze patterns, facial expressions, head movements, RRBs, cries and vocalizations, and on evaluating questionnaires, as well as medical data (e.g., imaging, molecular data) (Chaddad et al. 2021; Ghosh et al. 2021). A multimodal AI approach holds promise for early and accurate detection in the future (Mengi and Malhotra 2021). Although false positives and false negatives occur with AI, its rate of accurate diagnosis may outperform clinician evaluations. Thus, we are likely to see increased use of these technologies in the future.

Applied Behavior Analysis

Many consider autism a lifelong condition; however, a study by Ivar Lovaas in 1987 showed that preschool children who received more than 40 hours per week of one-on-one applied behavior analysis (ABA) early intervention for 2 years achieved much more favorable outcomes than a control group that received 10 hours or fewer per week of one-on-one ABA intervention. In fact, he reported that 47% of the children in the experimental group (40 hours per week) presented with average intellectual functioning, were placed in general education settings, and were indistinguishable from their nonautistic peers. Although this study has been critiqued, it led to schools, insurance companies, and other agencies providing many hours of one-on-one intervention for young children.

Although it has been commonly referred to as a scientifically based intervention for treating autism, ABA is not an intervention for autism but, rather, a term that has largely replaced the terms *behavioral psychology* or *behaviorism*, which also focused on observable events and teaching and modifying such events through operant and classical conditioning.

In the 1960s, Lovaas and colleagues began applying behavioral theory to teach language and to reduce the interfering behaviors of children with autism. Eventually, he described the intervention for autism as ABA. In addition, Lovaas et al. (1973) showed that parents were part of the solution, not the cause of autism—that is, they found that without parental participation and training, children were likely to lose the clinical gains they had made. This was in sharp contrast to interventions based on psychodynamic theories that viewed parents as the problem and separated their children from them.

ABA intervention carefully documents observable and measurable behaviors and breaks complex behaviors into small, manageable parts, with an emphasis on their consequences. The intervention that Lovaas and others developed in the 1960s was initially called *discrete trial training* and focused on presenting an instruction, waiting for a child response, then providing a consequence for that behavior (also described as "antecedent-behavior-consequence" or ABC) (Lerman et al. 2016; Lovaas et al. 1974).

Most autism centers and clinics report that some children do have optimal outcomes with ABA, although not all studies show as favorable a response as in the Lovaas (1987) study, in which almost half of the children responded optimally. Other studies suggest that with early intervention, almost 10% of children who clearly met the diagnostic criteria for autism in early childhood will eventually lose their diagnosis (Eigsti et al. 2023). As interventions improve through research, parents may be given more reason to be optimistic that children can improve dramatically with treatment.

Pivotal Response Treatment

Kanner (1943) recounted that the parents of his patients described some remarkable skills the children had acquired, such as the ability to repeat nursery rhymes, list the American presidents, recite prayers or poems, learn botanical names and composers' names, or recite the alphabet at an extremely early age, even before they were able to produce word combinations. This history is often overlooked, and these types of skills are too often unnoticed or ignored during assessment and in support and educational programs. However, these skills and strengths are exactly what we focused on when we developed pivotal response treatment (PRT), which greatly improved the learning curve and significantly reduced interfering behaviors during the teaching process.

PRT was initially published in 1987 as an intervention package (R.L. Koegel et al. 1987), although the individual components had been researched prior to that publication. The initial goal of PRT was to target the abstract notion of "motivation." That is, children with autism seemed unenthusiastic about attending ABA sessions, and many engaged in various strategies to avoid or escape them. The traditional ABA intervention principally began with focusing on eye contact and motor and sound imitation, with the notion that if the children could attend and imitate, they would make large gains. In addition, flash cards were used in a repetitive drill manner to teach vocabulary, language, and concepts. With these procedures, about half of the children with autism became verbal. However, half remained nonverbal, with no spoken words, despite having received intervention for verbal spoken communication.

Our initial PRT study included children with no spoken words who had been receiving traditional ABA therapy for many years without acquisition of first words. When we included the motivational components (specific procedures are described in detail in Chapter 2, "First Words and Word Combinations"), the children began to use verbal expressive words. Later research showed that most children (85%–95%) will learn expressive words with PRT if the intervention begins before age 5. Unfortunately, after age 5, only 20% of nonverbal children will learn expressive words, so targeting expressive verbal communication during the preschool years is extremely important. The initial PRT research focused on expressive spoken communication and therefore was termed the *natural language paradigm*. However, later publications showed that when specific "pivotal" areas were targeted, such as motivation, improvements in untargeted areas resulted; thus, the approach was renamed *pivotal response treatment*.

The steadily increasing rate of children being diagnosed with ASD, as noted by the Centers for Disease Control and Prevention (2024), has been accompanied by an increase in interventions targeting this population. Evidence-based interventions are particularly important because many procedures and treatments that have not been researched, or at least not at an acceptable level, are advertised to parents. Some involve risky procedures, others may cause discomfort to the child, and some are simply not effective. The need to accelerate the learning curve in many areas underscores the importance of implementing sound interventions. Although every person is individual, some interventions are more likely to be effective than others. For that reason, careful monitoring, regular data collection, and making adjustments to programs based on the data are vital. Before we dive into the details of PRT, Fred Volkmar, M.D., from Yale University, briefly discusses the importance of evidence-based interventions.

Evidence-Based Treatments, by Fred R. Volkmar, M.D., Yale University

Evidence-based treatments have a long history in medicine and now in fields such as psychology, speech-communication education, and so forth. The body of work came from a desire to provide services that were truly based on excellent scientific evidence rather than anecdote, and this is reflected in groups such as the Cochrane (www.cochrane.org) and Campbell (www.campbellcollaboration.org) collaboratives that provide periodic reviews of a range of techniques and practices.

In autism, the importance of interventions being evidence-based started with early work establishing that structured education was better than unstructured psychotherapy, and in the two decades after autism was first recognized, more research on treatments began to appear. By around 2000, several important reviews of effective treatments had been conducted, often using simple standards of effectiveness. For example, the National Research Council (2001) had a standard of one published peer-reviewed paper. Today, various standards have been adopted, but they typically are much more stringent, such as requiring replication of studies; double-blind, placebo-controlled studies; and/or meta-analyses. The standards chosen a priori do, of course, significantly impact what treatments/practices emerge as evidence-based.

Some treatments, such as ABA, do not lend themselves easily to the usual randomized controlled and double-blind trials but yield tremendous bodies of data supporting their effectiveness. Similarly, other models, such as statewide entitlement models, are not so easily studied in usual treatment effectiveness paradigms. With all the complexities and qualifications, a number of both model treatment programs and techniques have now emerged (see Steinbrenner et al. 2020 for a recent and excellent review), including model treatments such as PRT as well as other developmental approaches.

Ableism and Neurodiversity

Another area that has been discussed in the literature relates to ableism and neurodiversity. As the number of individuals diagnosed with ASD increased, the theoretical construct suggesting that neurological differences are a natural part of human diversity that should be accepted, embraced, and encouraged—rather than "cured"—began to emerge (Kapp et al. 2013). This neurodiversity movement, which has largely gained momentum online, has been active in promoting the strengths of individuals with ASD rather than viewing the condition as a disability, encourages active participation and feedback in research and intervention programs by neurodiverse individuals, and uses language that does not promote ableism (Bottema-Beutel et al. 2021). Primarily driven by a subgroup of autistic adults who are verbal, this movement has recommended identity-first language (IFL; e.g., *autistic person*) rather than person-first language (PFL; e.g., *person with autism*). Historically, disability-first language was used by researchers and practitioners prior to the 1980s, at which time parents began advocating for PFL, with the argument that many children could overcome the characteristics and that disability-first language was like saying "a broken-leg child." The nomenclature topic has been debated, and many parents and practitioners feel more comfortable with PFL, in contrast to the neurodiverse group, which prefers IFL.

The provision of intervention and support for young children has also raised some debate. Some in the neurodiverse group are opposed to autism interventions designed to "cure" or "normalize" a child, whereas others think that a "goodness of fit" for their socioemotional and physical environments should be considered. A strong and understandable motivation of this movement regarding treatment relates to the frequent use of punishment to decrease unwanted behaviors in early behavioral interventions and, reportedly, in psychodynamic treatments.

Sensitive and Inclusive Language

The neurodiversity movement also advocates for the reduction of ableist terms. Over the years, autism has been described in predominantly negative terms, with little emphasis on strengths and assets. The following suggestions for sensitive and inclusive language, adapted from my guidelines for the *Journal of Autism and Development* when I became editor and edited by associate editors, individuals on the autism spectrum, and others (Springer 2022), are suggested for psychiatrists and other practitioners.

> **IFL versus PFL.** If participants are adults and can understand, ask them to state their preference (congruent with reporters' and journalists' guidelines). If no preference is stated, use the more neutral phrase *on the autism spectrum*. Although preferences have shifted over the years, most autistic individuals seem to prefer IFL (Bottema-Beutel et al. 2021; Vivanti 2020), whereas many families and practitioners prefer PFL.

Nonautistic individuals. Refrain from using terms such as *healthy* or *normal*. Similarly, instead of *typical child* or *typical peer*, use *nonautistic children, children not diagnosed with a disability*, or the newer term *allistic*.

Patients' skills, abilities, and behaviors. Avoid using adjectives such as *high-functioning* and *low-functioning*. Instead, describe the characteristics of participants in detail across multiple domains.

Potential diagnosis. Avoid saying someone is *at risk* of developing autism. Use terms such as *an increased likelihood of being diagnosed with autism* or *correlated with a diagnosis of autism*.

Language skills. Rather than using vague terms such as *minimally verbal* or *nonverbal*, use specific standardized categories that relate to both age and expected linguistic development (L.K. Koegel et al. 2020). Could also use *nonspeaking* or *minimally speaking* (Botha et al. 2023).

Negative behaviors. In place of using vague terms such as *disruptive behaviors* or *autistic behaviors*, describe the specific behaviors.

Fatalistic language. Avoid terms that suggest autism is uniformly adverse and will lead to poor outcomes for families, individuals on the spectrum, or society. Discuss interventions that will be helpful to families, providers, and others while decreasing any conversation focused solely on weaknesses, problems, and deficits.

Strengths-based language. Include the strengths of the autistic person whenever possible, but do not minimize the challenges experienced by people on the autism spectrum and their families. Qualify those challenges, such as those associated with reduced educational or social opportunities or health care access for individuals on the spectrum, especially in cases in which individual or structural factors beyond autism are significant contributors.

Meaningful outcomes. Consider how any recommendations may result in quality-of-life improvements for the individual on the autism spectrum and/or their family.

Harmful or demeaning interventions. Interventions using procedures that cause pain or that increase the frequency of unwanted behaviors should not be used. Strengths-based approaches are increasingly accepted as best practice.

Other diagnoses. Avoid using *comorbid*. Use *coexisting* or *co-occurring*.

Comprehensive guidelines related to equity, diversity, and inclusion have been published by the American Psychological Association (www

.apa.org/about/apa/equity-diversity-inclusion/language-guidelines
.pdf).

Neurodiversity and Neurodiversity-Affirming Intervention: A Primer for Clinicians, by Zachary J. Williams, M.D., Ph.D., Vanderbilt University School of Medicine/Vanderbilt University Medical Center

The term *neurodiversity* has become quite popular in contemporary discourse about autism and developmental disabilities, although it also remains a frequently misunderstood and misapplied concept, particularly within clinical practice. Although a complete treatment of neurodiversity or its role in autism intervention is beyond the scope of this short section (interested readers are directed to Dwyer 2022, Gaddy and Crow 2023, Leadbitter et al. 2021, and Schuck et al. 2022), I aim to provide an overview of basic definitions and correct several common misconceptions about neurodiversity and neurodiversity-affirming interventions.

In and of itself, the concept of *neurodiversity* refers to the diversity of neurocognitive and/or sensory functioning that exists in the human population, encompassing all brains that are generally classified as "typical" or otherwise (Pellicano and den Houting 2022). In this sense, neurodiversity is akin to *biodiversity* (i.e., the diversity of species in an ecosystem) and remains an undeniable biological fact. However, the concept of neurodiversity also refers to the neurodiversity approach(es) (sometimes also called the "neurodiversity paradigm[s]"), a specific set of theoretical perspectives that reject the traditional medical model of disability and seek to depathologize many traits associated with autism and other neurodevelopmental conditions (Dwyer 2022). This again can be distinguished from the *neurodiversity movement,* a political activist movement that seeks to advance the rights and welfare of "neurodivergent" (i.e., neurocognitively atypical) individuals (Dwyer 2022; Ne'eman and Pellicano 2022).

As noted by Dwyer (2022), there is not one single neurodiversity approach/paradigm but, rather, a set of closely related approaches based on a shared set of foundational principles. A key tenet of these neurodiversity approaches is that disability is the product of an interaction between the characteristics of a disabled person and the environment around them. This interactionist model of disability rejects both 1) the strict *medical* model of disability, in which disability arises entirely from characteristics within a person (e.g., disease processes, pathological traits, impaired body functions) and 2) the strict *social* model of disability, in which disability is a social construct imposed on top of certain impairments by society, and the degree of disability is based entirely on how much these impairments are accommodated by society at large. A common misconception is that the neurodiversity approaches imply that autism and other neurodevelopmental conditions are not disabilities but instead are mere differences. Although the neurodiversity approaches may dispute claims that these conditions (or traits associated with them) are inherently dysfunctional, pathological, or undesirable, they still always acknowledge that such conditions remain sources of disability for neurodivergent individuals (typically because of interactions between individual traits/characteristics and the environmental/social context) (Ne'eman and Pellicano 2022). Thus, the neurodiversity approaches are more about viewing certain disabilities (and notably not all disabilities) within a value-neutral and non-pathologizing framework than about denying that they are disabilities in the first place.

Neurodiversity approaches also diverge from the medical model in terms of their goals for disability-focused interventions, which under the medical model seek to "fix," "cure," or "normalize" the disability or pathological traits to the greatest extent possible (Haegele and Hodge 2016). Because neurodiversity approaches view disability as an interaction of individual traits and the environment, they specifically oppose the goals of curing or normalizing the disabled person as ends in themselves (Dwyer 2022), instead focusing on promoting person-environment fit in order to reduce functional impairment (Lai et al. 2020). Notably, this does not mean that the neurodiversity approach only supports environmentally targeted interventions (as with the strong social model [Haegele and Hodge 2016]) or that it is incompatible with intervention entirely; rather, as I and others have argued elsewhere (Pantazakos and Vanaken 2023; Schuck et al. 2022), a number of behavioral interventions (including naturalistic developmental behavioral interventions and several psychotherapy modalities) can be made to theoretically align with the neurodiversity approach when practiced according to "neurodiversity-affirming" clinical principles. Although this theoretical alignment does not guarantee that such interventions are practiced or that their practitioners are working in alignment with the neurodiversity approach or the goals of the neurodiversity movement, it does allow for neurodiversity-affirming intervention to exist as more than just a buzzword or marketing term.

Pantazakos and Vanaken (2023) noted three key principles that make an intervention neurodiversity-affirming: 1) engaging in participatory research and therapy, 2) resisting normalization and respecting consent, and 3) implementing environmental interventions (Chapman and Botha 2023). The first of these, engaging in participatory research and therapy, requires that autistic stakeholders be involved in the intervention as more than passive recipients. Neurodiversity-affirming interventions are often co-created or modified with input from autistic or neurodivergent community members to ensure that the content is respectful and that the treatment prioritizes outcomes meaningful to autistic/neurodivergent people.

The second principle, resisting normalization and respecting consent, ensures that the goals of treatment are in line with neurodiversity approaches—that is, they do not view autism or other neurodivergent traits as pathologies to be cured or normalized. By respecting the patient's consent (or assent, in the case of those who cannot consent for themselves) to treatment, providers employing neurodiversity-affirming interventions allow the recipient to be maximally in control of the treatments they receive and continually assess social validity (Schuck et al. 2022). As clarified by Pantazakos and Vanaken (2023), this does not mean that neurodiversity-affirming intervention requires uncritically affirming an autistic or neurodivergent person's cognitions, emotions, or behaviors, particularly if they are ultimately deleterious to that person's well-being. Pushing against the patient's "default modes" and challenging them is indeed a part of neurodiversity-affirming therapy, but such strategies should be continuously subject to reevaluation to ensure they generate outcomes that are meaningful to the patient and remain justified (Pantazakos 2025).

Third, the principle of implementing environmental interventions urges clinicians to be open to the possibility that a given problem or area of disability is best addressed not by individual change but by an environmental change or an accommodation of difference by others.

Naturalistic developmental behavioral interventions such as PRT are some of the early intervention techniques most aligned with the neurodiversity approaches, although the ways they are currently practiced in most settings do not typically fully conform to all three neurodiversity-affirming clinical principles. For a more thorough exploration of how these interventions can be aligned with the neurodiversity approaches, see Schuck et al. (2022).

Summary

Over time, great changes have occurred in the hypothesized causes of and ensuing treatments for ASD. Early parental causation theory has long been dismissed, and parents are now viewed as critically important for child gains. Parent participation is an integral part of treatment programs. Although psychiatrists and other providers and consultants may consider some areas not important to address, verbal autistic adults report that, despite the challenges of socialization, they yearn for friendships and relationships across the lifespan. Creating inclusive environments where socialization and social communication can be supported is essential (Black et al. 2024). Focusing on the strengths of people on the autism spectrum is critical for assessment and intervention. PRT strategies that focus on individual strengths and preferences can be instrumental in providing support within rewarding contexts.

References

American Psychiatric Association: Diagnostic and Statistical Manual of Mental Disorders, 2nd Edition. Washington, DC, American Psychiatric Association, 1968

American Psychiatric Association: Diagnostic and Statistical Manual of Mental Disorders, 3rd Edition. Washington, DC, American Psychiatric Association, 1980

American Psychiatric Association: Diagnostic and Statistical Manual of Mental Disorders, 3rd Edition, Revised. Washington, DC, American Psychiatric Association, 1987

American Psychiatric Association: Diagnostic and Statistical Manual of Mental Disorders, 4th Edition. Washington, DC, American Psychiatric Association, 1994

American Psychiatric Association: Diagnostic and Statistical Manual of Mental Disorders, 5th Edition. Arlington, VA, American Psychiatric Association, 2013

American Psychiatric Association: Diagnostic and Statistical Manual of Mental Disorders, 5th Edition, Text Revision. Washington, DC, American Psychiatric Association, 2022

Asperger H: Die "autistischen psychopathen" in kindesalter. Arch Psychiatr Nervenkr 117:76, 1944

Bettelheim B: Love Is Not Enough: The Treatment of Emotionally Disturbed Children. New York, Free Press, 1950

Bettelheim B: The Empty Fortress: Infantile Autism and the Birth of the Self. New York, Simon & Schuster, 1967

Black MH, Kuzminski R, Wang J, et al: Experiences of friendships for individuals on the autism spectrum: a scoping review. Rev J Autism Dev Disord 11:184–209, 2024

Bohm HV, Stewart MG, Healy AM: On the autistic spectrum disorder concordance rates of twins and non-twin siblings. Med Hypotheses 81(5):789–791, 2013 24055096

Botha M, Hanlon J, Williams GL: Does language matter? Identity-first versus person-first language use in autism research: a response to Vivanti. J Autism Dev Disord 53(2):870–878, 2023 33474662

Bottema-Beutel K, Kapp SK, Lester JN, et al: Avoiding ableist language: suggestions for autism researchers. Autism Adulthood 3(1):18–29, 2021 36601265

Centers for Disease Control and Prevention: 2000–2020 Data and Statistics on Autism Spectrum Disorder Prevalence. Atlanta, GA, Centers for Disease Control and Prevention, May 16, 2024. Available at: https://www.cdc.gov/autism/data-research/?CDC_AAref_Val=https://www.cdc.gov/ncbddd/autism/data.html. Accessed November 6, 2024.

Chaddad A, Li J, Lu Q, et al: Can autism be diagnosed with artificial intelligence? A narrative review. Diagnostics (Basel) 11(11):2032, 2021 34829379

Chapman R, Botha M: Neurodivergence-informed therapy. Dev Med Child Neurol 65(3):310–317, 2023 36082483

Cruz S, Zubizarreta SCP, Costa AD, et al: Is there a bias towards males in the diagnosis of autism? A systematic review and meta-analysis. Neuropsychol Rev 2024 [Epub ahead of print]

Dwyer P: The neurodiversity approach(es): what are they and what do they mean for researchers? Hum Dev 66(2):73–92, 2022 36158596

Eigsti IM, Fein D, Larson C: Editorial perspective: another look at "optimal outcome" in autism spectrum disorder. J Child Psychol Psychiatry 64(2):332–334, 2023 35772988

Gaddy C, Crow H: A primer on neurodiversity-affirming speech and language services for autistic individuals. Perspect ASHA Spec Interest Groups 8(6):1220–1237, 2023

Gau SSF, Chou MC, Chiang HL, et al: Parental adjustment, marital relationship, and family function in families of children with autism. Res Autism Spectr Disord 6(1):263–270, 2012

Ghosh T, Al Banna MH, Rahman MS, et al: Artificial intelligence and internet of things in screening and management of autism spectrum disorder. Sustain Cities Soc 74:103189, 2021

Haegele JA, Hodge S: Disability discourse: overview and critiques of the medical and social models. Quest 68(2):193–206, 2016

Kanner L: Autistic disturbances of affective contact. Nerv Child 2(3):217–250, 1943

Kapp SK, Gillespie-Lynch K, Sherman LE, et al: Deficit, difference, or both? Autism and neurodiversity. Dev Psychol 49(1):59–71, 2013 22545843

Klaiman C, White S, Richardson S, et al: Expert clinician certainty in diagnosing autism spectrum disorder in 16–30 month olds: a multi-site trial secondary analysis. J Autism Dev Disord 54(2):393–408, 2024

Koegel LK, Bryan KM, Su PL, et al: Definitions of nonverbal and minimally verbal in research for autism: a systematic review of the literature. J Autism Dev Disord 50(8):2957–2972, 2020 32056115

Koegel RL, Schreibman L, O'Neill RE, et al: The personality and family-interaction characteristics of parents of autistic children. J Consult Clin Psychol 51(5):683–692, 1983 6630681

Koegel RL, O'Dell MC, Koegel LK: A natural language teaching paradigm for nonverbal autistic children. J Autism Dev Disord 17(2):187–200, 1987 3610995

Lai M-C, Anagnostou E, Wiznitzer M, et al: Evidence-based support for autistic people across the lifespan: maximising potential, minimising barriers, and optimising the person-environment fit. Lancet Neurol 19(5):434–451, 2020 32142628

Leadbitter K, Buckle KL, Ellis C, et al: Autistic self-advocacy and the neurodiversity movement: implications for autism early intervention research and practice. Front Psychol 12:635690, 2021 33912110

Lerman DC, Valentino AL, LeBlanc LA: Discrete trial training, in Early Intervention for Young Children With Autism Spectrum Disorder. Edited by Lang R, Hancock TB, Singh NN. New York, Springer, 2016, pp 47–83

Loomes R, Hull L, Mandy WPL: What is the male-to-female ratio in autism spectrum disorder? A systematic review and meta-analysis. J Am Acad Child Adolesc Psychiatry 56(6):466–474, 2017 28545751

Lovaas OI: Behavioral treatment and normal educational and intellectual functioning in young autistic children. J Consult Clin Psychol 55(1):3–9, 1987 3571656

Lovaas OI, Koegel R, Simmons JQ, et al: Some generalization and follow-up measures on autistic children in behavior therapy. J Appl Behav Anal 6(1):131–165, 1973 16795385

Lovaas OI, Schreibman L, Koegel RL: A behavior modification approach to the treatment of autistic children. J Autism Child Schizophr 4(2):111–129, 1974 4479842

Lu J, Wang Z, Liang Y, et al: Rethinking autism: the impact of maternal risk factors on autism development. Am J Transl Res 14(2):1136–1145, 2022 35273718

Mengi M, Malhotra D: Artificial intelligence based techniques for the detection of socio-behavioral disorders: a systematic review. Arch Comput Methods Eng 29(4):1–45, 2021

National Research Council: Educating Young Children With Autism. Washington, DC, National Academy Press, 2001

Ne'eman A, Pellicano E: Neurodiversity as politics. Hum Dev 66(2):149–157, 2022 36714278

Pantazakos T: Neurodiversity and psychotherapy: connections and ways forward. Couns Psychother Res 25(1):e12675, 2025

Pantazakos T, Vanaken G-J: Addressing the autism mental health crisis: the potential of phenomenology in neurodiversity-affirming clinical practices. Front Psychol 14:1225152, 2023 37731874

Pellicano E, den Houting J: Annual research review: shifting from "normal science" to neurodiversity in autism science. J Child Psychol Psychiatry 63(4):381–396, 2022 34730840

Rimland B: Infantile Autism: The Syndrome and Its Implications for a Neural Theory of Behavior. New York, Appleton-Century-Crofts, 1964

Schuck RK, Tagavi DM, Baiden KMP, et al: Neurodiversity and autism intervention: reconciling perspectives through a naturalistic developmental behavioral intervention framework. J Autism Dev Disord 52(10):4625–4645, 2022 34643863

Springer: Journal of Autism and Developmental Disorders: Submission Guidelines. London, Springer Nature, 2022. Available at: https://www.springer.com/journal/10803/submission-guidelines#Instructions%20for%20Authors_Editorial%20procedure. Accessed November 6, 2024.

Steinbrenner JR, Hume K, Odom SL, et al: Evidence-Based Practices For Children, Youth, and Young Adults With Autism. Chapel Hill, NC, The University of North Carolina at Chapel Hill, National Clearinghouse on Autism Evidence and Practice Review Team, 2020

Vashisth S, Chahrour MH: Genomic strategies to untangle the etiology of autism: a primer. Autism Res 16(1):31–39, 2023 36415077

Vivanti G: Ask the editor: What is the most appropriate way to talk about individuals with a diagnosis of autism? J Autism Dev Disord 50(2):691–693, 2020 31676917

Wing L: Asperger syndrome: a clinical account. Psychol Med 11(1):115–129, 1981 7208735

Wing L: The relationship between Asperger's syndrome and Kanner's autism, in Autism and Asperger Syndrome. Edited by Frith U. New York, Cambridge University Press, 1991, pp 93–121

2

First Words and Word Combinations

Early Diagnosis

An early autism diagnosis can lead to early referrals for support programs. In this chapter, I discuss social communication and other areas that parents and professionals should be aware of when obtaining an early diagnosis.

Prior to the onset of spoken words, children whose language is coming in at expected milestones demonstrate several prelinguistic communicative behaviors that are social in nature, including eye contact, pointing, joint attention (in which the child purposefully shares attention between an item and another individual), responsiveness to their name being called, smiles, gestures, and social vocalizations. Regarding spoken communication, also referred to as "expressive words and language," babbling that begins around age 6 or 7 months generally turns into first words around age 12 months, and by 18 months, children usually have a vocabulary of up to 20 distinct words. These are largely words to which they are frequently exposed by their care providers. Most first lexicons include "mama" and "dada," some animal sounds, "hi," and "bye-bye" (although these vary slightly across cultures, with some having a larger variety of relatives' titles).

Children with autism develop their first words at a slower rate, resulting in smaller vocabularies, and the nature of their lexical profiles differs from that of children who are developing language typically. They tend to use more words relating to food, drink, and actions (e.g., "cookie," "juice," "stop," "eat," "tickle"), whereas typical language learners tend to use more social words and verbs (e.g., "see," "kiss," "look") (Haebig et al. 2021). In short, children with autism are more likely to use communication for requests for items and actions and less frequently for social attention and interaction.

Although parents may report noticing challenges with prelinguistic social, play, sensory, and repetitive behaviors, a child's lack of first words or loss of early words is generally the catalyst for parents seeking professional help (Guinchat et al. 2012). Thus, for some families, it may be close to a child's second birthday when parents express concern about their child's development. However, some children later diagnosed with autism will demonstrate early word use and even apparently advanced language acquisition, such as repeating nursery rhymes, the alphabet, counting, and so on. This great heterogeneity results in a wide age range for when children are first diagnosed. Other variables, such as socioeconomic status, being female, being from an ethnic minority, and lacking a stable primary care physician may also delay a diagnosis.

Although autism spectrum disorder (ASD) can be reliably diagnosed by 18 months of age, the average age at diagnosis is later than 3 years for boys and 4 years for girls. In fact, before age 3, less than two-thirds of parents of children with autism have reported a concern to their child's doctor, and fewer than one-fifth of children with autism have received a diagnosis (Zablotsky et al. 2017). It has been shown that parents who express concern about their child's prelinguistic differences are more likely to get an earlier diagnosis. Providers should ask parents about these early preverbal behaviors, particularly because children diagnosed by age 2½ exhibit greater improvements than those diagnosed later, when cognitive and treatment hours are held constant (Gabbay-Dizdar et al. 2022). Thus, early diagnosis and intervention are critical. Table 2.1 lists some of the prelinguistic signs of ASD that parents and clinicians should look out for.

Table 2.1 Prelinguistic signs of autism spectrum disorder

Lack of an orienting response when name is called

Low levels of babbling, including canonical babbling (in which infants repeat consonant-vowel sounds, such as "mamamama" and "dadadada")

Little eye contact

Lack of pointing, which should begin around age 9–12 months

Lack of joint attention, including following the gaze of a parent, which should begin at age 4–6 months

Low responsiveness to early social games (e.g., peek-a-boo)

Few smiles and low affect (sometimes infants will smile when tickled or thrown in the air but will do so less frequently in social situations)

Low levels of gesture use (e.g., reaching upward to be picked up, waving, nodding head)

Playing repetitively with objects, such as repeatedly turning on and off a light, spinning the wheels of a toy car, or placing objects near the eye to examine with altered visual input

Exhibiting repetitive movements, such as repetitive hand flapping or examining their own hands for periods of time

Under- or overreaction to sensory input (e.g., textures, noises), such as loud sounds, tight clothing, or clothing tags

---

Case Example: Frankie

During Frankie's 1-year checkup, his mother reported that he was a quiet and easy baby. He ate well and had met all his first-year motor milestones as expected. However, as he neared his first birthday, she noticed that he did not appear interested in social engagement. Although a few spinning toys interested him, he did not seem interested in common games such as "peek-a-boo" and "so big," despite repeated attempts to engage him. Furthermore, he became upset whenever she put his shoes on him, and he would try to remove them. He made a few vowel sounds, but they were not directed toward her, and she reported that she had never heard him attempt to say any consonants or words.

Case Example: Jamie

Jamie was a fussy baby who began humming songs by age 7 months. Her parents heard a few word attempts that disappeared by her first birthday. When they called her name, she did not look up, nor had she begun to point or to follow a point. They could elicit a smile if they tickled her but reported that no other activities resulted in a smile.

Case Example: Dexter

Dexter's parents noted nothing unusual about his motor, verbal, or social milestones during his first year of life. By age 1 year, he had a good vocabulary with clear articulation. However, they reported that he took little interest in others' activities, preferring to stare at their ceiling fan for hours. If they turned the fan off, he engaged in a meltdown that could last for hours until they relented and turned the fan back on.

These children all eventually received a diagnosis of ASD, but not until well after their second birthdays. Frankie's mother reported that she had hesitated to tell her doctor about her concerns out of fear of "getting a diagnosis," and each time the doctor did not express his own concerns, she breathed a great sigh of relief. Jamie's pediatrician suggested a hearing test and indicated that if Jamie had acquired no words by age 18 months, he would refer her to a speech and language specialist. Dexter's pediatrician indicated that most milestones were being met at expected times, and therefore a "wait and see" approach was best.

These patterns of a later diagnosis are common because children without autism vary in their word acquisition. Infant temperaments also vary widely. However, activities and programs exist that can be implemented during the first years of life for infants and young children who are showing characteristics of autism, and addressing parental concerns and social and communicative issues at the earliest point in time—even before first words are expected—is advantageous for the child. This leads us to the important issue of early diagnosis and prognosis.

The onset of first words by 24 months of age leads to better outcomes, and, in general, evidence has shown that children with higher cognitive and language skills will have a more favorable prognosis—that is, children who enter intervention programs with higher skills will exit those programs with higher skills (L.K. Koegel et al. 2019). After 5 years of age, a smaller percentage of children who are completely nonverbal will acquire spoken words as a primary mode of communication. Again, intervention at the earliest point in time is critical. Although many reports have been made of "late talkers" who excelled in life, it is always difficult to get a clear picture of a child's development from retrospective reports years later. Most children can improve their delayed communication (and other areas) significantly if their parents are given the proper tools, so early intervention with parent participation is extremely valuable. However, some of the interventions available for children diagnosed with autism or showing early characteristics of autism are adult-driven and therefore not enjoyable for the child. The clear and common avoidance behaviors demonstrated by children on the autism spectrum who received the most effective treatments that were available in the 1960s and 1970s (and unfortunately are still being used in some centers today) led us to explore techniques that would be enjoyable for young children. Because the children appeared to demonstrate a lack of "motivation," we began a research line focused on strategies that would improve children's motivation to engage and respond (and to do so correctly). We hypothesized that a motivated child would not demonstrate behaviors used to escape and avoid these teaching situations.

First, a little background. As described in Chapter 1 ("Autism Overview and the Development of Pivotal Response Treatment"), pivotal response treatment (PRT) was first called the *natural language paradigm* because our early studies focused on teaching verbal words to children who were nonverbal. This is known as a "top-down" approach. Once children reach an age at which they should have a good-sized lexicon, expressive first words are targeted. This is important because many behaviors can be targeted later, but spoken communication is less likely to be acquired if first words are not targeted and learned early on. As mentioned earlier, only a small percentage of nonverbal children learn spoken expressive communication after age 5, so there is some time pressure on this. Children may never catch up if they are enrolled in intervention programs that begin teaching early nonverbal communication before the children achieve their first words—a "bottom-up" approach. However, when intervention starts at a higher level (i.e., targeting spoken words), many early behaviors fall into place. For example, when teaching first words using PRT, the important areas of joint attention and social engagement emerge without needing to be specifically taught (Bruinsma 2004; Ebrahim 2019; Vismara and Lyons 2007).

Learned Helplessness

Before we discuss how to teach first words, a theoretical background is helpful for understanding the key concepts behind PRT. The notion of targeting motivation as a key area was based on the theory that children on the autism spectrum often develop *learned helplessness*. Learned helplessness develops when individuals do not connect their behavior with the outcome of the behavior, resulting in lower levels of responding or a lack of responding altogether. Early studies related to this theory were conducted with animals that, after being restrained under painful conditions, stopped attempting to escape the pain (Seligman 1972), even after the restraint was removed and escape was possible. Later studies conducted with humans showed that when confronted with difficult situations, such as repeatedly failing to solve a problem or being confronted with a loud noise that could not be stopped, participants eventually stopped trying or showed significantly longer response times. Thus, when such lack-of-control situations repeatedly occur, whether real or perceived, they can reduce individuals' motivation and persistence and may result in depression, anxiety, and other mental health conditions. In other words, when the behavior and the consequences of the behavior are not linked, the result is less motivation to attempt to control the situation and a general failure to learn what actions are necessary to control the outcome.

Children with autism who have difficulty with certain tasks may not be rewarded for their attempts, or they may receive noncontingent rewards that can lead them to stop trying. For example, parents may inadvertently communicate for their child or may provide desired items without expecting communication; a teacher may finish putting a child's jacket on so that he is not late for the bus; a peer may ignore a child's attempt at socialization because her communication is not clear; or parents may feed their child themselves after his food repeatedly drops off his fork. In these situations, the child is not connecting their behavior with the consequence. Repeated and frequent exposure to such situations causes the child to respond more slowly or less often and, in some cases, to stop responding at all. To reverse this cycle, teaching procedures are put in place that focus on the "pivotal" area of motivation. Targeting pivotal areas, rather than individual areas, results in more widespread changes in untargeted areas. Logically, if a child is motivated, they will engage and respond more, with faster learning.

The following section discusses the PRT teaching components that are specifically designed and have been shown to be effective for improving learners' motivation. When these strategies are incorporated into teaching, learners respond faster, produce more correct responses, show improved levels of engagement and higher affect, and engage in lower levels of interfering and disruptive behaviors.

Motivational Components of Pivotal Response Treatment

Child Choice

The first critical component of PRT is child choice. For children learning their first words, the toys and activities that they prefer are incorporated into their treatment sessions. Choice may be assessed by observing the child, interviewing others, and using preference assessments in which various items are presented to the child. Those items in which the child expresses interest are selected for use during sessions.

Because preferences may change from session to session and even minute to minute, it is important to remain vigilant to such changes. Similarly, a child may choose a preferred food or activity, but after filling up on that snack or engaging in that activity for a while, they may lose their preference for it, at which time another preferred item or activity should be incorporated.

Case Example: Danny

> Danny enjoys watching the light being turned on. Therefore, his parents decide to prompt him to say "on" before turning on the light.

Please note that using an intense interest, even if it is not common, is desirable for teaching first words. Using an intense interest during intervention does not cause an increase in the behavior at other times (Baker 2000; Baker et al. 1998; Charlop et al. 1990).

Case Example: Erin

Erin loves car rides. Her parents prompt her to say "go" whenever she wants to go for a ride. After this word becomes routine, and she can say it readily, they prompt "key" and "open" while on the way to the car. This further expands her vocabulary, using her preferred interest in car rides.

Case Example: Jose

Jose's favorite food is potato chips. Although his parents prefer that he eat a healthy diet, they decide to use "chip" to prompt his first word because this seems to be the most motivating item for him. Once he can say "chip," they expand this to "open" before opening the chip container, and then pause expectantly for him to request a chip spontaneously without the modeling. Gradually increasing the number of different words Jose says before getting his favorite food keeps his response level and motivation high while thinning out the number of chips he eats. (Note: small pieces of chips can also be used instead of a whole chip to increase the number of responses before the child satiates.)

Case Example: Xavier

Xavier cried and whined a good part of the day, particularly when others tried to engage with him or presented a learning activity. He saw a speech therapist twice a week and had some daily hours of in-home applied behavior analysis (ABA). However, his excessive crying made the sessions of little to no benefit. We decided to teach him the word "bye" so he would have a tool to terminate an interaction or situation that he wanted to avoid or escape. After just two short sessions, Xavier began to replace his crying with "bye." Once he made the connection between using a word and the positive and desired outcome of the word, he began to engage for longer periods of time before saying "bye." Over time, he began to use words frequently and consistently.

Natural Rewards

Using child choice fits nicely with providing natural rewards or natural consequences. Traditional ABA assessed items that were rewarding for the child and provided them as a consequence for giving correct responses. Often, these were food treats and were unrelated to the child's behavior. However, our team's research (R.L. Koegel and Williams 1980) showed that if the reward was naturally connected to the behavior being taught, children with autism showed rapid acquisition of the behavior, compared with a very slow or lack of acquisition if there was no connection. For example, in contrast to rewarding the child with a treat after labeling a picture of a ball, the child is provided with an actual ball to play with after saying "ball."

Case Example: J.J.

J.J. repetitively watches cartoons. Her favorite is a *Peppa Pig* episode, "Birthday Surprise," which she replays over and over again. Her parents decide to prompt her to say "on" as a first word, every time she wants to watch the cartoon. As soon as she says "on," her parents immediately turn on the cartoon and let her watch it as a natural reward.

Case Example: Pedro

Pedro spends hours each day placing a ball at the top of a toy ramp and watching it roll down. When the ball gets to the bottom, an adult picks it up and prompts him to say "ball." Right after he makes a verbal attempt at the word "ball," the adult lets him enjoy watching it roll down as a natural reward.

Case Example: Beto

Beto likes his father to throw him up in the air and reaches both arms up to his dad when he wants to be thrown. Instead of responding to the nonverbal cue, his dad prompts Beto to say "up" before picking him up and tossing him in the air as a natural reward for his verbalization.

Case Example: Aram

Aram pulls his mother's hand and leads her to items he wants, including the door handle when he wants to go outside. Aram's mother prompts him to say "come" instead of simply pulling her along. As soon as he makes a verbal attempt at saying the word "come," she immediately goes where he is taking her as a natural reward for saying "come."

Reward Attempts

Often, new behaviors are difficult for children on the autism spectrum, and their attempts are not rewarded. In addition, some of the outdated techniques recommend a strict shaping paradigm in which only responses that are as good as—or better than—the previous response are rewarded.

For first words, rewarding any and all true attempts is important, even if the attempt is not a perfect production of the adult word (R.L. Koegel et al. 1988). When rewarding attempts, however, it is important that only "true" attempts be rewarded. Sometimes a child is not trying at all—looking away, engaging in other off-task behaviors—but emits a correct or somewhat correct response. In PRT, *trying* is what is most important. If a child is not really trying but instead is making a series of responses that do not appear to be intentional or is sifting through various sounds until they accidentally hit the correct one, it is important to not provide the natural reward. Because the goal of PRT is motivation, the child who is not motivated should not be rewarded. However, if the child is making a good attempt, their response should be rewarded, even if it is not entirely correct.

Case Example: Bridget

> Bridget is learning to say her first words and is infatuated with balloons. She especially enjoys when adults blow up a balloon and let it go so she can watch it fly around the room. Some of the first words that the team decides to prompt are "balloon," "blow," and "go." Bridget says "ba" for "balloon" when her parents prompt the word, after which they enthusiastically bring a balloon. She also says "bo" for "blow" and "ga" for "go." After each of these attempts, her parents model the correct word and then follow through with the activity, even though her words are not perfectly pronounced.

Case Example: Michael

> Michael is 4 years old and has not yet spoken an expressive verbal word. During our initial sessions, he stared into space when prompted to say a word, appearing to not understand what was being asked of him. However, we found that during snacks, he would utter sounds while eating. We began by modeling a word, such as "cracker," waiting until he made a sound, then providing the cracker to him right after the sound. Shortly thereafter, Michael made the connection between

the vocalization and the sound and regularly began making vocalizations for his favorite snack. This was the beginning of his acquisition of many additional words.

Case Example: Jin

Jin loves to have bubbles blown. He is learning his first words and pronounces the word "baba" and sometimes only "ba" just before they are blown. Because he is in the fragile initial word learning stage, each and every verbal attempt is rewarded immediately, even if it is one or two syllables that only partially resemble the adult pronunciation.

Case Example: Ben

Ben was having a tough time learning the power of words and did not seem to understand the connection between verbally requesting an activity and the positive outcome of that request. He especially enjoyed when adults blew a harmonica and often spontaneously brought it to an adult to blow. After several weeks of unsuccessfully prompting the word "harmonica" and "blow," we decided to prompt him just to blow (not saying the word, just simply blowing out air), which he easily picked up. After that first attempt, we prompted animal sounds for other favorite toys. Simplifying the adult word by using a sound seemed to be helpful in getting those first words started.

Case Example: Jeremy

Jeremy was 19 months old and was showing characteristics of autism, including a lack of smiles, no pointing, little response to his name being called, and infrequent babbling. However, he imitated a raspberry sound whenever his mother modeled it. To teach him that words (or sounds) have meaning, we began prompting the raspberry sound, then immediately gave him his favorite fruit. Within a few minutes, he was consistently making the sound to get a blueberry.

Intersperse Acquisition and Maintenance Tasks

Most children on the autism spectrum have multiple areas that would benefit from support. It is tempting to drill those challenging areas so that the child gets a lot of opportunities to practice. However, this may be discouraging for the child and lead to lower responsiveness and fewer correct responses. In contrast, when new (acquisition) tasks are interspersed with previously acquired (maintenance) tasks, greater responsiveness and faster learning occur (Dunlap 1984). Thus, if a program just drills, drills, drills on new tasks without including already mastered tasks, the child is likely to progress more slowly. Perhaps this is behavioral momentum, in which a series of easy tasks followed by a difficult one creates a tendency to persist with the more challenging one because the child is being rewarded more frequently. Although it may seem counterintuitive that a child will learn faster when easy and difficult tasks are mixed rather than by being presented with non-mastered activities, this is the case for children on the autism spectrum.

Case Example: Douglas

Fifth grader Douglas is learning his multiplication tables. The teacher has given him worksheets with dozens of multiplication problems. When he sees the teacher handing out the sheets, he looks visibly upset and works at a snail's pace. To improve his motivation, we mixed addition and subtraction problems, which are easy for him, with the multiplication problems. Now Douglas completes several that he knows and takes a stab at the multiplication problems. When the easy and hard math problems are interspersed, he gets more multiplication problems correct and more worksheets completed.

Case Example: Jenna

Jenna has learned a few words ("more," "drink," and "open"), which she says consistently. Because she is almost 4 years old, her speech therapist is prompting additional words. Initially, the speech therapist only prompted the new words, which were emerging extremely slowly. However, after the therapist began interspersing the learned words with new words, Jenna's vocabulary blossomed.

Often, children understand that different words convey different meanings after they can consistently say at least 10 different words. Before learning an initial lexicon, they will overgeneralize the few words they know. Thus, acquiring those new words is important, but repetitively asking the child to use new words without interspersing the mastered ones can result in slower learning. After children have acquired about 50 words, they usually start combining words.

Case Example: Jake

> Jake could use a lot of single words, at least 60 reliably and consistently, so his new goal was to combine words. Combining words was tough for Jake, so the adults interspersed two-word prompts with one-word prompts.

Although some children easily move to two words, particularly if they consistently use each word, others have more difficulty learning to combine words. Thus, interspersing this acquisition task of combined words with the single words was helpful in reducing Jake's frustration.

Task Variation

Task variation is also helpful for improving motivation. Instead of presenting a single task over and over until the child reaches mastery, research shows that varying the tasks results in better outcomes (Dunlap and Koegel 1980). Furthermore, combining task variation with interspersed maintenance tasks has an even greater positive effect. Children also show more enthusiasm, interest, and happiness during the teaching sessions when their tasks are varied.

Case Example: Lucas

> Lucas is learning to spell words. His teacher mixes writing the words with spelling them out loud and lets Lucas play teacher and "test" her on the words. She also gives him an opportunity to pick some words that he would like to learn how to spell (child choice) and includes words that he already has mastered (interspersal).

Case Example: Liam

> Liam is learning how to write letters. His teacher has selected his favorite items (choice) and is prompting him to write the first letter of the item. She mixes this activity with opportunities for verbal communication and simply identifying letters to vary the task. She provides the desired item right after each response as a natural reward.

Case Example: Christopher

> Christopher began hitting and pushing other children. A careful examination of this behavior indicated that he was attempting to

interact with his peers but had not learned appropriate ways to interact socially. He was able to say short sentences, so his mother prompted him to say "Wanna play?" instead of using aggression. She also varied this by prompting him to hand a toy to another child, say "your turn" and "my turn," and to push other children on the swing. Quite rapidly, Christopher began using his prosocial behaviors, which resulted in children playing with him rather than avoiding him.

Teaching Communication

As discussed, our early PRT studies focused on communication, in particular verbal words. First words depend on the child's interests and motivations. Consequently, using the PRT motivational components greatly increased the number of children who could learn to use verbal words as a primary mode of communication. Items and activities that the children enjoy will be their first words. If a child is in a program in which the provider or adult decides what first words a child should learn, regardless of the child's interest, progress will be slow. It is critical to follow the child's lead and to look for preferred items and interests to begin prompting first words. However, a small portion of children remain who, even with early intervention, do not learn verbal communication. For these children, augmentative and alternative communication (AAC) may be warranted. Several factors must be considered before settling on teaching these methods, including the child's age, communicative potential for spoken communication, previous program(s), training, coordination, and parental interest.

Augmentative and Alternative Communication or Verbal Communication

Deciding if and when to start a child with AAC has been discussed widely in the literature. Various AAC systems are available, ranging from signs and gestures (referred to as "unaided" because they do not require additional materials) to more complex ("aided") systems that can be used on electronic devices. Although AAC used either as a supplement or by itself can be helpful for children with complex communication needs, there are several considerations.

More research is needed in this area, but some have argued that combining AAC with intervention may be helpful in facilitating first words with some language programs (Pope et al. 2024). However, data show that minimally verbal and nonverbal children ages 4 and younger who are diagnosed with autism may not learn first words more rapidly if an AAC picture program is introduced prior to targeting expressive words (Schreibman and Stahmer 2014). In addition, most parents report that they prefer to focus on teaching verbal communication over AAC when their children are young (Schreibman and Stahmer 2014). Some programs, particularly those that are more structured and do not contain motivational components, have a lower likelihood of helping children become verbal; thus, the type of program in which the child has been participating should be evaluated. However, gestures that are easily understandable by others can be helpful prompts while teaching first words.

A challenge with studies assessing the effectiveness of AAC in early language use is that most parents, clinicians, and teachers will (and should) reward any word or word attempt, so it is nearly impossible to compare the effects of AAC alone with a verbal-only approach and to conclude that AAC facilitated verbal communication. Furthermore, it has been well documented that when AAC is taught at school or in a clinic, most parents do not follow through with an AAC system at home because they understand their children's needs through nonverbal communication, they find using AAC to be cumbersome, and they may not have adequate training on how to effectively use AAC (Suhr et al. 2024). Often, the time spent teaching an augmentative system could be used for teaching verbal communication, and once an AAC device is being used, a child may get frustrated and exhibit meltdowns if they cannot use the device when verbal communication is prompted later.

Other reported barriers to AAC include the need for training (both professionals and parents), which should be implemented across settings and providers, but this is not always the case. Parents report that many AAC devices are not easy to learn to use; their children often do not see the value of training to use them and simply use them improperly. Some AAC devices are expensive and not affordable for families. Parents also report that it can be difficult integrating AAC into daily life with busy schedules, parenting demands, caring for other children, challenges when extended family visits, and the limitations their child has with social interactions. Sometimes natural interactions suffice for understanding their child's needs, and parents can interpret facial expressions, body movements, pointing, eye gaze, and so on (Berenguer et al. 2022). Unfortunately, most AAC systems are abandoned within a year.

The facts that most nonverbal children with autism (85%–95%) will learn to use verbal spoken communication as their primary mode of communication (L.K. Koegel 2000) and that parents of young children prefer a focus on verbal communication (Schreibman and Stahmer 2014) have led us to begin prompting verbal words using the PRT motivational procedures. There is no hard and fast rule for when to move to AAC if a child is not acquiring verbal communication; although some 2- and 3-year-old children with autism will emit their first words within one or two PRT sessions, others sometimes take considerably longer, even up to a year or two.

After age 5, however, if a child is completely nonverbal, it is very difficult to teach first words. There are various hypotheses as to why verbal communication may be more difficult to acquire after age 5 (Newport et al. 2001). Some have suggested that there are "critical ages" for language learning. Others believe that children simply learn to communicate effectively without words. Whatever the reason, intensive early intervention for verbal communication is critical because the success rate is higher with children younger than 5. Then, after age 5, if the child has received a motivational program without success, AAC may be a viable option. It is also important to use motivational components when starting an AAC system so that the child can make the connection between these types of communicative behaviors and the message they communicate. Parents of children with autism report that their children may view computerized AAC devices as toys to play with, rather than as a communicative tool (Berenguer et al. 2022). In addition, we occasionally prompt clear gestures to accompany verbal communication if a young child is difficult to understand, or if the child becomes frustrated because they do not have enough words yet to convey their meaning.

Case Example: Tony

After a few months of being prompted to say verbal words, 3-year-old Tony began to make some word attempts, but his vocabulary was too small for specificity. He often led his parents to the kitchen, pulling them by the hand, and made some attempt at requesting food but became upset when they could not guess what he wanted. To reduce his frustration, we made him a picture board with photographs of his favorite foods. Now, when Tony takes his parents to the kitchen and says "Eeee" for "eat," they get out the picture board, and he points to the specific item he wants.

Case Example: Adam

Adam began using verbal words around age 3, after more than a year of prompting. His initial words were only consonant-vowel sounds and vowels, such as "o" for "open," "da" for both "drink" and "dada," "e" for "eat," and "ma" for both "more" and "mama." He tended to mix the words and run through all his newly learned sounds when he wanted something, so it was almost impossible to understand what he was trying to say. Teaching him a few simple gestures with the word, such as having him put his hand to his mouth when he was hungry or having him pick up an imaginary cup and make a drinking gesture when he was thirsty, made his word attempts clear.

Case Example: Patrick

Patrick, a young adult, came to us with no verbal words and no AAC system. Although several programs had reportedly been attempted, his providers indicated that they had been ineffective. We tried having Patrick exchange a picture of a favorite item printed on an index card for that item, but he did not respond. Once we enlarged the picture of the item to 8" × 10", he was able to exchange the picture with accuracy. It was unclear whether he had a visual or attention challenge, but this manipulation solved the problem.

Case Example: DeShawn

DeShawn was highly echolalic when he came to us at age 6. While focusing on decreasing his echolalia and teaching more functional verbal communication, we began noticing that when he verbally requested an item or activity, such as saying "ride" when he wanted to go someplace, he became frustrated if his parents were unable to guess *where* he wanted to go. Adding pictures to their phones that he could swipe through provided DeShawn with an opportunity to be more specific with his communication. These useful pictures were also used to prompt his words, thereby improving his verbal communication.

For some individuals, teaching them to exchange an actual item rather than a representation of the item can be helpful for the initial use of an AAC system. For example, one adolescent was able to learn to hand us a cup from an array of items when he was thirsty.

Facilitated Communication

Along with the right to communicate is the right to be sure one is communicating for oneself (Shane 1994). Some programs involve significant prompting of individuals to communicate using letter boards or keyboards, but the resulting communication has been scientifically shown to be that of the facilitator and not the autistic individual. Tragically, dozens of individuals with autism made unfounded accusations of rape, incest, and inappropriate sexual acts, resulting in these individuals being removed from their homes and charges being filed against their parents. Although these claims were eventually found to be false, they caused the families suffering and trauma, and in most cases, the autistic individuals were deprived of seeing their parents during the investigative process. Professionals have also been fired from their jobs when they were falsely accused of sexual crimes. Not surprisingly, these false allegations led to many lawsuits.

Many programs today use letter boards and typing programs, and for the individuals who can access communication this way, we encourage these types of AAC. However, given that every individual has a right to communicate their *own* needs, wants, feelings, beliefs, and thoughts, it is critical that objective assessments be put in place to ensure the *individual* is communicating and not the facilitator. This can be done in several ways. For example, the facilitator can be shown a different item or picture or asked a different question when the child is asked to write the name of the item or the answer. The facilitator can be asked to look away while supporting the child so that they do not inadvertently guide the individual to specific letters. The facilitator can be asked to leave the room while an item is shown to the individual or a question is asked, and then the facilitator can support the individual upon returning. Using systematic tests to ensure the autistic individual is the true author of any messages is essential.

Prompting First Words

When prompting first words, we recommend that the word alone be modeled for the learner. Saying too many words in the prompt may confuse the child. For example, if a child wants to go outside and the adult says, "Oh, I see you are by the door. Do you want me to open it for you?" the child may not be clear on the precise word to use. Alternatively, if the adult says "open," then pauses for the child to repeat the word, it is clear what is expected. Once a child has a good vocabulary, it is a good idea to model a few extra words, but only after the child has enough words to understand that each word has its own label.

Creating Spontaneity

Once a child can imitate a model by repeating words that are verbally presented, it is time to fade the prompts to encourage independent and spontaneous word use. Adults can provide a pause (also called a *time delay*) with an expectant look, rather than modeling a word, to encourage the child to use the word without needing the model. Some children require more gradual prompt fading, such as giving the first sound of the word before pausing. A word is not considered to be "learned" until the child can say it independently across many settings. If a child only says "cup" for the red one used at home but does not label any other cups, the concept has not been acquired. It is important to make sure that the adults fade their prompts as quickly as possible (but systematically) so that the child does not become dependent on the adult's model.

Extra Prompts for First Words

Although PRT is effective for most children, a small percentage do not seem to understand the connection between using expressive words and the positive outcomes of these words. For these children, the following additional techniques may be helpful to suggest to parents and providers. Remember, you will still want to use the PRT motivational strategies with these additional supports.

- **Improve attention**. Research on nonresponders to traditional PRT shows that often it is a lack of attention to the verbal model that interferes with verbal communication. If a child appears to be giving full attention to the desired item and not to the verbal model, an orienting cue can be used. Orienting cues may be a high-five, tickle, or gesture that gains the child's attention and can be used immediately before the label of the item is presented. These orienting cues must be individualized; therefore, it is important to try different orienting cues until an effective one is discovered (R.L. Koegel et al. 2009).
- **Use carrier phrases**. *Carrier phrases* are familiar verbal routines, such as "ready, set, go" or "one, two, three," that can be used just before providing a desired action. Once the child is anticipating

the upcoming action, pausing before the last word and giving the child an opportunity to say "go" or "three" can be helpful. These types of prompts can help the child anticipate what is coming and serve as a cue for the child to complete the last word of the carrier phrase.

- **Incorporate songs.** Many children enjoy music and songs. Leaving off the last word of a familiar song and waiting with an anticipatory look can be a prompt for the child to complete the song. Using music may tap into different areas of the brain and can facilitate first words for some children.
- **Use sounds or words in the child's repertoire.** Nonverbal children often make sounds or will repeat words out of context (also referred to as *echolalia*). If these sounds or echolalic words are paired with real items, the child often learns the connection of words representing items or actions.

Case Example: Mick

Mick enjoyed the handful of musical toys his family owned and became extremely excited when an adult turned on the music. He focused so intently on the toy that he seemed oblivious to anything else that was going on around him and did not repeat the modeled label of the word. To get his full attention off the toy and onto the name of the toy, the adults sang a few musical notes. Once his attention was gained by singing "la, la, la, la, la" in the tune of "Crocodile Rock," the word "music" or "on" was modeled, and he began to repeat the word.

Case Example: Nick

Nick had been receiving PRT for several months but had not yet started saying first words or making word attempts. Nick's favorite activity was swinging, in which he could engage for hours. Instead of simply pushing him, his parents began saying "one-two-three" and then pushing him. After several days, they noticed that he became very animated when they started counting, so they paused before saying "three," at which time Nick began to excitedly say "three." This connection was the first step of a rapid increase in his vocabulary.

Case Example: Miranda

Miranda did not use words to communicate, but her mother noticed that when she sang to Miranda, the child effortlessly finished the last word of the stanza if her mother paused and gave an expectant look, whether it was "E-I-E-I-O," "Twinkle, Twinkle Little Star," or "The Wheels on the Bus." Armed with this information, Miranda's mom began making up short little songs during everyday activities, and after some time with a song, she would pause before the last word. Miranda's vocabulary grew rapidly using these musical prompts.

Case Example: Eleanor

Eleanor was nonverbal; however, her parents reported that she consistently repeated the word "bubble" when watching her most preferred video, in a section where bubbles were blown. Upon observation, we noted that she clearly repeated the word "bubble" every time bubbles appeared. Interestingly, when we brought out a real bottle of bubbles and prompted her to say "bubble," she remained silent. However, when we began blowing bubbles at the same time they appeared in the video, she said "bubble," and we were able to transfer the word to the actual item. Following acquisition of this first word, her vocabulary blossomed.

Intelligibility

Some children emit their first words with perfect articulation, even with later-developing sounds. Others begin with word attempts that are far from the adult pronunciation of the word. Sometimes words will become more intelligible with repeated use, and other times a sound or syllable may need to be slightly stressed to prompt the child to be clearer. For example, if a child says "oh" for "open," the adult may need to say "pen" a little louder, so the child attends to the second syllable. Similarly, if a child says "da" for "done" when wanting to finish an activity, the "n" can be emphasized. Other PRT techniques can be used with individual phonemes during natural activities once the child has a large repertoire of words, which produces more rapid acquisition than traditional speech therapy for articulation (R.L. Koegel et al. 1998).

Generally, children will have about 50 single words in their repertoire before beginning to combine words. If these single words are unintelligible, the word combinations may be even less intelligible, so a focus on articulation with single words may be helpful. A speech-language specialist may be helpful in guiding parents on how to improve articulation. Again, our research has shown that PRT can be used to improve articulation; instead of drilling the child, using preferred objects, task variation, and natural rewards to target sounds in words during natural interactions results in higher levels of positive affect, faster learning of targeted sounds, and greater generalization of newly learned sounds (R.L. Koegel et al. 1998).

Spontaneous Words

Once a child is consistently responding to verbal model prompts, encourage parents and other adults to provide a time delay or pause to encourage spontaneous use of communication without a model. If a child does not consistently use a word across settings without a model, the word is not considered to be acquired. Sometimes it is helpful to suggest that a parent ask an open-ended question such as "What do you want?" or "What should we do?" to encourage spontaneous use of spoken words. Parents can also look at the child expectantly before giving the child a desired item or engaging in a desired activity to encourage spontaneous word use. Finally, for some children, it is helpful to gradually fade the prompt by saying just the initial sound or syllable of a word. We do not want the child to become frustrated or discouraged; thus, the model prompt (i.e., the word) should be faded slowly and gradually so the child still connects the word with the desired outcome. This way, the child will not become prompt-dependent on an adult to help them with communication.

Word Combinations

Many children on the autism spectrum will begin using word combinations independently. Others who exhibit echolalia—repeating a word, phrase, or sentence just after (*immediate echolalia*) or some period of time after it was heard (*delayed echolalia*)—may use these echolalic utterances in appropriate contexts. For example, you may hear them say "open door" or "more milk" without special instruction, just as a typical language learner will do. Other children continue using single words until special instruction is provided. If a child has a good repertoire of intelligible words, care providers should begin recasting the child's utterance. *Recasting* means that an adult will say the same word the child uses but will add a word or two. For example, if the child says "open" independently while standing by the door, the adult may recast that word by saying "open the door," or if a child says "juice," the parent can say "more juice" or "more juice, please." This way, the child is exposed to the longer utterance using the preferred word.

If a child does not start combining words without support, selecting two words that are meaningful and prompting the child to combine them can be helpful. For example, if a child requests "car" and knows the colors, I might prompt "red car" and give the red car as a natural reward after both words are produced. Similarly, if a child says "open" and knows the word "door," "open door" can be prompted. Be aware that children use unique word combinations. If a child's only sentences are "I want X," "I want Y," and "I want Z," it is likely that this phrase is memorized and is serving the purpose of a single word. The child has not learned the rules of syntax and that words can be combined in novel ways. Thus, making sure that words are combined and used flexibly and in different contexts is important.

Once a child is combining words regularly, language growth is better if adults do not simplify their utterances. Using "motherese" or omitting important words in the sentence is not helpful once the child is combining words. For example, if the adult says, "Put in box" rather than "Put it in the box," the child's language is not likely to progress as quickly as when the grammatically correct phrase or sentence is used. Again, when teaching a first lexicon, we want to keep it simple by modeling the single word, but once the child begins to combine words, using incorrect grammar by leaving out articles or other key words is not recommended for the most favorable language outcomes.

Summary

Most children diagnosed with ASD will learn to use verbal communication if support and considerable opportunities across contexts are provided during the preschool years. Using the PRT motivational components accelerates the acquisition of first words compared with adult-driven approaches (R.L. Koegel et al. 1987). AAC systems are available for the small percentage of children who do not acquire verbal words in the preschool years despite good intervention programs, ample opportunities, and coordination across settings. Speech-generating devices that are handheld or on a portable computer can be used. Signs and gestures can be very helpful either alone or with the verbal word for prompting verbal communication and with first words for children with intelligibility issues. The use of AAC strategies is highly recommended if the child is older than 5 years and is completely nonverbal despite efforts at verbal communication. The PRT motivational techniques can be used in tandem with the AAC system. However, because

AAC strategies are not generally used in the home or over time, their usefulness for the family and child warrants consideration.

The high likelihood of nonverbal preschool-age children acquiring first words and more complex communication using the PRT motivational components corroborates the benefits of early intervention with a strong focus on expressive verbal communication. PRT procedures should be used frequently in everyday contexts, and the individual's goals, procedures, and expectations should be coordinated across everyone with whom they interact, in order to produce the most favorable outcomes.

References

Baker MJ: Incorporating the thematic ritualistic behaviors of children with autism into games: increasing social play interactions with siblings. J Posit Behav Interv 2(2):66–84, 2000

Baker MJ, Koegel RL, Koegel LK: Increasing the social behavior of young children with autism using their obsessive behaviors. J Assoc Pers Sev Handicaps 23(4):300–308, 1998

Berenguer C, Martínez ER, De Stasio S, et al: Parents' perceptions and experiences with their children's use of augmentative/alternative communication: a systematic review and qualitative meta-synthesis. Int J Environ Res Public Health 19(13):8091, 2022 35805750

Bruinsma YE: Increases in the Joint Attention Behavior of Eye Gaze Alternation to Share Enjoyment as a Collateral Effect of Pivotal Response Treatment for Three Children With Autism. University of California, Santa Barbara, 2004

Charlop MH, Kurtz PF, Casey FG: Using aberrant behaviors as reinforcers for autistic children. J Appl Behav Anal 23(2):163–181, 1990 2373653

Dunlap G: The influence of task variation and maintenance tasks on the learning and affect of autistic children. J Exp Child Psychol 37(1):41–64, 1984 6707578

Dunlap G, Koegel RL: Motivating autistic children through stimulus variation. J Appl Behav Anal 13(4):619–627, 1980 7204282

Ebrahim MTES: Effectiveness of a pivotal response training programme in joint attention and social interaction of kindergarten children with autism spectrum disorder. Psycho-Educational Research Reviews 8(2):48–56, 2019

Gabbay-Dizdar N, Ilan M, Meiri G, et al: Early diagnosis of autism in the community is associated with marked improvement in social symptoms within 1–2 years. Autism 26(6):1353–1363, 2022 34623179

Guinchat V, Chamak B, Bonniau B, et al: Very early signs of autism reported by parents include many concerns not specific to autism criteria. Res Autism Spectr Disord 6(2):589–601, 2012

Haebig E, Jiménez E, Cox CR, et al: Characterizing the early vocabulary profiles of preverbal and minimally verbal children with autism spectrum disorder. Autism 25(4):958–970, 2021 33246365

Koegel LK: Interventions to facilitate communication in autism. J Autism Dev Disord 30(5):383–391, 2000 11098873

Koegel LK, Bryan KM, Su P, et al: Intervention for nonverbal and minimally verbal individuals with autism: a systematic review. Int J Pediatr Res 5(2):056, 2019

Koegel RL, Williams JA: Direct versus indirect response-reinforcer relationships in teaching autistic children. J Abnorm Child Psychol 8(4):537–547, 1980 7462531

Koegel RL, O'Dell MC, Koegel LK: A natural language teaching paradigm for nonverbal autistic children. J Autism Dev Disord 17(2):187–200, 1987 3610995

Koegel RL, O'Dell M, Dunlap G: Producing speech use in nonverbal autistic children by reinforcing attempts. J Autism Dev Disord 18(4):525–538, 1988 3215880

Koegel RL, Camarata S, Koegel LK, et al: Increasing speech intelligibility in children with autism. J Autism Dev Disord 28(3):241–251, 1998 9656136

Koegel RL, Shirotova L, Koegel LK: Brief report: using individualized orienting cues to facilitate first-word acquisition in non-responders with autism. J Autism Dev Disord 39(11):1587–1592, 2009 19488847

Newport EL, Bavelier D, Neville HJ: Critical thinking about critical periods: perspectives on a critical period for language acquisition, in Language, Brain, and Cognitive Development: Essays in Honor of Jacques Mehler. Edited by Dupoux E. Cambridge, MA, MIT Press, 2001, pp 481–502

Pope L, Light J, Laubscher E: The effect of naturalistic developmental behavioral interventions and aided AAC on the language development of children on the autism spectrum with minimal speech: a systematic review and meta-analysis. J Autism Dev Disord 2024 38848009 [Epub ahead of print]

Schreibman L, Stahmer AC: A randomized trial comparison of the effects of verbal and pictorial naturalistic communication strategies on spoken language for young children with autism. J Autism Dev Disord 44(5):1244–1251, 2014 24272416

Seligman ME: Learned helplessness. Annu Rev Med 23(1):407–412, 1972 4566487

Shane HC (ed): Facilitated Communication: The Clinical and Social Phenomenon. San Diego, CA, Singular Publishing Group, 1994

Suhr M, Bean A, Rolniak J, et al: The influence of classroom context on AAC device use for nonspeaking school-aged autistic children. Int J Speech Lang Pathol 26(3):434–444, 2024 37395393

Vismara LA, Lyons GL: Using perseverative interests to elicit joint attention behaviors in young children with autism: theoretical and clinical implications for understanding motivation. J Posit Behav Interv 9(4):214–228, 2007

Zablotsky B, Colpe LJ, Pringle BA, et al: Age of parental concern, diagnosis, and service initiation among children with autism spectrum disorder. Am J Intellect Dev Disabil 122(1):49–61, 2017 28095057I

3

The Importance of Initiations

In this chapter, I discuss methods that psychiatrists and health care providers can use to encourage parents to promote child-initiated interactions and to expand the functions of communication. Evidence shows that the bulk of language used by children on the autism spectrum consists of requests (e.g., "I want juice") and protests (e.g., "no" or "stop"), rather than the wide variety of communicative functions necessary for communicative competence. I describe specific strategies for teaching other functions of communication, including question-asking, commenting, play initiation and entering play, attention-seeking strategies, and assistance-seeking strategies, using the motivational pivotal response treatment (PRT) procedures, as well as simple strategies to assess patients' needs during office visits.

An important (and maybe critical) assessment that should be made during an initial office visit or consultation relates to the functions of the child's communication. If PRT is started during the preschool years, most children will learn expressive spoken communication and will use this method as their primary mode of communication. However, regardless of the intervention program used, many children on the autism spectrum primarily use requests to communicate their needs and wants. These may be single words, such as "cookie," or sentences, such as "I want drink" or "Can I have car, please?" Some children even develop words to convey protests, such as "all done," "bye-bye," or "no," when they want to terminate an activity or interaction. In contrast, children who develop communication without challenges exhibit a variety of communicative functions in their repertoires, which include social initiations. In fact, social questions often are evident in a typical language learner's first lexicon. For example, a child whose language is developing typically may point to an item and say "this" or "that" as a simple request for information. This is a rudimentary form of the question "What's this?" or "What's that?" after which a parent or adult will label the item for the child. Consequently, children develop large vocabularies using this child-initiated strategy. It is both social and information-seeking. In contrast, analyses of language samples of children on the autism spectrum show that these types of initiations are rare or nonexistent (L.K. Koegel et al. 2022; Wetherby 1986).

Long-Term Outcomes

In a small longitudinal study, we retrospectively analyzed videotapes to understand prognostic indicators that may be associated with more positive outcomes in children with autism (L.K. Koegel et al. 1999). The literature suggests that a verbal IQ of around 60 or above at a young age and the presence of verbal communication by age 5 are associated with more favorable outcomes; however, many children with these characteristics are not able to live independently, gain meaningful employment, develop relationships, and engage in other important social and community activities later in life. Reviewing other variables that may be relevant to improved outcomes in children who are verbal, we analyzed archival data, including standardized testing and video recorded interactions of children with their parents during the preschool years, ranging from 2 years and 7 months to 3 years and 10 months. Specifically, we analyzed the outcomes of adolescents and young adults who should have had a good prognosis according to their standardized tests and language abilities. The results of these analyses suggested that children who initiated interactions with their parents had more favorable outcomes than children who did not. Children who rarely or never initiated interactions with their parents as preschoolers had different outcomes, including lower language levels, fewer social interactions, lower likelihood of going to college or holding jobs, and lower community involvement compared with those who verbally or nonverbally initiated interactions by bringing toys to their parents, pointing out items, or engaging interactively in other ways.

Given these data, we implemented a second study that focused exclusively on teaching initiations to young children. Following this intervention, the children demonstrated more favorable outcomes, including a greater number of reported friends, more involvement in social events, more inclusion in mainstream classes, and greater academic achievement (L.K. Koegel et al. 1999). After this preliminary study, which focused on the long-term outcomes of 10 children, we conducted additional studies using controlled, single-subject designs and randomized clinical trials to further assess the importance of initiations. Specifically, we focused on teaching verbal initiations in the form of question-asking. Our research showed improved outcomes, both short- and long-term, for children who were taught to initiate questions. As in our first study, children who did not initiate interactions or use questions at baseline had improved outcomes when our intervention program focused on teaching initiations. Many interventionists teach targeted areas, such as vocabulary, prepositions, pronouns, and verbs, without considering the child initiations that may lead to independent learning of these linguistic structures. We emphasize the importance of teaching initiated communication, such as question-asking, within the curriculum because it appears to be "pivotal" in producing widespread gains (R.L. Koegel et al. 2014).

Assessment

The absence or a low frequency of initiations may be present across the lifespan, even among autistic individuals with advanced language skills. For children, the presence or absence of initiations can be assessed during office visits by having the parent and child interact naturally and asking the parent not to begin (i.e., initiate) any interactions, just to respond or complete any interactions initiated by the child. It is sometimes helpful to ask the parents to record a short video of their child with a sibling or peer during natural play interactions.

To assess language in everyday situations, a language sample can also be collected. To do this, have the parent and child interact naturally and ask the parent to encourage the child to talk as much as possible. Generally, it is helpful to collect at least 50 child utterances, but for children who talk infrequently, this may take too much of the appointment time, so fewer utterances can be analyzed. The data collected during language samples are helpful to understand how much the child talks relative to the communicative partner, how the child uses language (e.g., whether they just make requests or use language socially), the functions of the child's communication (e.g., whether they ask questions), and other variables such as rate of speaking, prosody, and so on.

Another great method for assessing whether initiations are present in verbal children, adolescents, or adults is by presenting "leading statements" during social conversation. For example, the examiner might say, "I had a great weekend," "I'm excited about my upcoming vacation," or "I'm feeling a little tired today." After the leading statement, the speaker should pause to provide the individual an opportunity to ask a question. If there is a long pause with no response, the individual responds with a single word or short phrase (e.g., "Oh, really" or "Wow!"), or they bring the topic back to their own interests without responding to the leading statement, teaching question-asking is recommended.

Case Example: Angel

Three-year-old Angel came in for an assessment. He had a good-sized vocabulary and could combine words to make short sentences. During the first 10 minutes of the office visit, we asked the parent to play with Angel and try to get him to talk as much as possible while we wrote down everything that he said in order to identify appropriate goals. A close inspection of his utterances showed that his communication was exclusively used for requests and protests. He could use a variety of words and short phrases for desired items, such as "Pick me up, please," "Give me juice," "I want candy," and "Bye-bye" or "All done" when he wanted to terminate an interaction. However, he did not ask questions or use other functions of communication. Thus, we recommended beginning a question-asking program with him.

Case Example: Ivan

Ivan was in his early twenties and excelled in college. His only concern was that he did not have friends, and although he dated occasionally, he rarely secured a second date. An assessment of his conversation revealed that he did not ask any questions during social interactions. We purposely provided pauses in the conversation during the assessment to give him an opportunity to ask questions, but these only resulted in periods of long, awkward silence. His lack of question-asking was interfering with his ability to develop close relationships.

Case Example: Cameron

Cameron was a teenager who expressed an interest in making more friends. During the office visit, he was very responsive and quite interesting discussing his knowledge of travel, math, and the Harry Potter series. Throughout his social conversation, he seldom asked questions, even when leading statements were provided, such as "I love the Harry Potter characters, too." In such instances, he often responded with "Oh!" and then went on to describe his favorite character. Although he was interested in social interaction, the number of his utterances expressing an interest in the communicative partner was so low that the conversation was more of a monologue than a back-and-forth interaction.

Strategies for Teaching Initiations

If a child is combining words and making requests but is not asking many or any questions, recommending a program to improve this area is warranted. When recommending that a family work on question-asking, stress that the PRT motivational components be included. Child-initiated questions often lead to linguistic demands, so with the PRT motivational components incorporated from the outset, the child begins by being naturally rewarded after asking a question. We generally teach question-asking in the order that types of questions are acquired developmentally by children without language delays. The following are step-by-step procedures for teaching question-asking.

Question: "What's That?"

A simplified version of "What's that?" (or "What's this?" depending on which a parent uses with their child) is the first question that emerges in typical language learners. Children at the one-word stage will simplify this utterance and ask simply "Dis?" or "Dat?" after which parents and other adults label the item for the child. This type of question helps children develop a large and diverse vocabulary (L.K. Koegel et al. 1998). Furthermore, it is social and child-initiated, reversing the cycle of adults needing to arrange and instigate teaching-learning interactions.

Pre-Teaching

Begin by gathering an opaque bag, some of the child's favorite items, and various neutral items that the child has not yet learned to label. If you are unsure about what items the child can or cannot label, determine this by asking the child "What is this?" while holding each item up. Intersperse these items with questions such as "What is this?" about the favorite items so the child is motivated to respond. Do not assume the child knows how to label everyday items; we have been surprised when some children have not picked up the labels of items to which they are frequently exposed, such as soap, underwear, hammer, nail, and so on.

Teaching

- *Step 1: Prompt the child to ask the question.* Start by placing only their favorite items in the opaque bag. This step is a motivational step only, so it does not matter if the child knows the label or not. The point is to help them make the connection between this new communicative structure and the positive outcome that will ensue after asking the question. Prompt the child to ask, "What's that?" This may be accomplished by simply saying, "Ask me, 'What's that?'" It may take several prompts before the child repeats the question. Some children are used to being asked this question, so they will try to answer rather than ask. Others may repeat the whole prompt ("Say, "What's that?""); if they do repeat, just say, "What's that?" as a prompt.
- *Step 2: Label the item.* After the child asks, "What's that?" immediately pull out a favorite item, label it, and have the child repeat the label.
- *Step 3: Provide a natural reward.* Immediately after the child has labeled the item, give it to them as a natural reward.
- *Step 4: Fade the verbal prompt.* Once a child begins repeating the question, provide a pause to allow them time to ask the question without the verbal prompt. Sometimes it is helpful to shake the bag a bit to get the child's attention. Repeat steps 2 and 3 after the child asks the question spontaneously.
- *Step 5: Add neutral items.* Once the child is independently and consistently asking the question with favorite items, begin gradually adding the neutral items that the child does not already label. Begin with every fourth trial, then every third, and so on

until the child is asking "What's that?" about the neutral items. Repeat steps 2 and 3 whenever the child asks the question.

- *Step 6: Fade the bag.* Now the opaque bag can be faded. Place the items on the table. At this point, the child should be able to ask, "What's that?" about items in the natural environment.

Case Example: Jason

Three-year-old Jason was able to request items using short sentences, but his parents had never heard him ask a question. We began teaching him to ask, "What's that?" using the motivational procedures just described. After a few months of intervention, Jason was requesting something from his mother, but she did not understand what he wanted. He began to become frustrated, then stopped, pointed to a box of granola bars on the top shelf, and asked, "What's that?" When his mother responded, "Granola bars," he firmly stated, "I want granola bars." Having question-asking in his repertoire was instrumental in reducing his frustration and subsequent meltdowns.

Case Example: Monica

Monica was 3½ years old and had not yet asked a question. We began using the motivational procedures to prompt her to ask, "What's that?" but she would not respond. A careful analysis showed that she would willingly repeat the label of any item she could see, such as "pencil," "paper," "shirt," "hair," and so on, but would not repeat items she could not see, such as "sky," "moon," or an abstraction such as "What's that?" To overcome this issue, we started asking her to repeat only "that" while pointing to the opaque bag. Once she was repeating "that," we added the "What's," and soon she was asking "What's that?" during the teaching activity. Shortly after, she began using the question at school and at home.

Case Example: Braden

Braden was 5 years old and was able to combine words. He knew his colors, could count, and had a good vocabulary, but he did not use any questions in his communication and was frequently unresponsive to adults if they asked him something that was not of high interest to him. Knowing that he was fascinated by planes, we put several small toy planes in the opaque bag as an initial step. When we first prompted him to ask, "What's that?" he responded by labeling the item we pointed to, saying "bag" instead of repeating the question. When we let him peek in the bag, he began to respond with "plane" instead of "What's that?" For so many years, adults had asked him, "What's that?" and now he had difficulty learning that he could ask the question himself. Instead of going straight to the prompt of the question, we asked him to repeat a few words: "Can you say 'table'?"; "Can you say 'chair'?"; "Can you say 'pencil'?" and then moved to the prompt "Can you say 'What's that?'" which helped him to repeat the question.

This procedure, which included the motivational components of child-preferred items (provided initially) along with natural rewards, was effective in teaching "What's that?" to children on the autism spectrum who had never used questions in their communication. Our community data also showed that the children spontaneously began to ask the question at home and at school without the need for additional teaching in those environments. However, language samples indicated that the acquisition of "What's that?" did not generalize to the use of other questions. Therefore, we began teaching the children a second question that is acquired developmentally: "Where is it?"

Please note that the first question generally takes the longest to acquire. Subsequent questions are often emitted by the child during the first teaching session.

Question: "Where Is It?"

Once a child has acquired "What is it?" acquisition of the second question, "Where is it?" is usually accomplished much faster, often during the first session. Again, to maintain the child's motivation, we use preferred items, which are then provided as a natural reward (L.K. Koegel et al. 2010). In addition to this utterance being child-initiated, the end goal is for the child to acquire prepositions as a result of using this question. Around 2 years of age, the prepositions *in, on,* and *under* begin to be used. By age 3 and beyond, additional prepositions seen in typical language users include *in front of, in back of, next to, beside, between,* and *behind.*

Pre-Teaching

Begin by gathering the child's favorite items. If you are unsure whether the child uses various prepositions, determine this by placing desired objects in different locations and asking the child where they are before providing access to the items. Sometimes collecting a language sample or asking parents can be helpful for understanding which prepositions the child uses.

Teaching

- *Step 1: Hide the child's favorite items.* The items should be hidden in locations that will include the targeted prepositions (e.g., in, on, under, behind, in front of, between, next to).
- *Step 2: Prompt the child to ask the question "Where is it?"* It can be helpful to provide a leading statement before the prompt to provide context. For example, "I hid the red car! Ask me, 'Where is it?'"
- *Step 3: Label the location.* After the child asks, "Where is it?" provide the location using the target preposition (e.g., "It's under the pillow," "It's behind the chair," "It's in the cup"). Be sure not to point to the item, or the child may use the nonverbal cue instead of listening to the answer.
- *Step 4: Have the child label the location.* Before the child can take the item, prompt the child to repeat the label of the location to practice expressive use of the preposition.
- *Step 5: Provide the natural reward.* Give the child an opportunity to play with the favorite item once it has been retrieved from the correct location. This can be repeated using various locations.
- *Step 6: Fade the verbal prompt.* After the child responds well to the prompt, provide a time delay or motion in a questioning way to prompt spontaneous use of the question.

Question: "Whose Is It?"

Many children on the autism spectrum have difficulty reversing pronouns. They often say, "You want water" or "Pick you up" when they mean "I want water" or "Pick me up." The following procedures are effective in teaching a self-initiated question that focuses on the acquisition of pronouns.

Pre-Teaching

Gather the child's favorite items and a variety of neutral items that belong to you. Neutral items can be items clearly associated with you but not of high desire to the child, such as pens, pencils, wallet, purse, books, and so on.

Teaching

- *Step 1: Prompt the question.* Place the desired items and the neutral items in front of the child. Hold up a desired item and prompt the child to ask, "Whose is it?"
- *Step 2: Respond.* After the child asks the question "Whose is it?" respond with "It's yours."
- *Step 3: Prompt the pronoun reversal.* Prompt the child to reverse the pronoun and say, "It's mine" or "Mine!"
- *Step 4: Provide the natural reward.* Give the desired item to the child.
- *Step 5: Fade the verbal prompt.* Provide a delay to give the child an opportunity to ask, "Whose is it?" without a verbal prompt.
- *Step 6: Teach "It's yours."* Once the child asks, "Whose is it?" without prompting and reverses the pronoun without prompts, intersperse a few of the neutral items. That is, after the child is successful with reversing the pronoun and can respond with "Mine," hold up one of the neutral items and after the child asks, "Whose is it?" say, "Mine!" and prompt the child to say, "Yours!" You can then set that item aside and return to the preferred item. Interspersing the desired items once you begin adding the neutral items will keep the child responding and interested.

This same procedure can be used to teach the possessive, such as Mommy's, Daddy's, sister's, brother's, and so on, if the child needs practice with possessives. Again, items clearly associated with a particular person can be included. These should be interspersed with favorite items to keep the child's motivation high.

Question: "What's Happening?" and "What Happened?"

Around age 2, most typical language learners have several verbs in their repertoires and have mastered the *-ing* ending. Also around this time, children begin to use the past tense, and by age 3 or 4, they have mastered most past-tense verbs, with the exception of some irregular verbs. Many children on the autism spectrum use a limited number of verbs and may need assistance with conjugation, *-ing* endings, and past tense. Expanding the variety of verbs and conjugations a child uses can also be accomplished through targeting child initiations. If the child does not use either the *-ing* ending on verbs or the past tense, the following are steps to teach this using a child initiation. Obtaining a language sample or asking the child what someone is doing or just did will help you assess whether they use the *-ing* and past-tense verb endings. Parents may also be helpful in reporting which verbs and verb endings they have heard the child use.

Pre-Teaching

Begin by gathering pop-up books with topics around the child's interests.

Teaching

- *Step 1: Set up your opportunity.* Manipulate a tab of the pop-up book. If the target goal is -ing endings, continue to manipulate the tab during step 2. If the child's goal is to use past tense, stop manipulating the tab after a few seconds.
- *Step 2: Prompt the question.* Prompt the child to ask, "What's happening?" or "What happened?"
- *Step 3: Respond.* Respond to the child's question, making sure to include a verb with the proper ending, such as "The snake is slithering" or "The car bounced."
- *Step 4: Prompt the child to repeat the verb ending.* Listen carefully for the *t* or *d* sound at the end of regular past-tense verbs. If the child exaggerates the sound a bit initially, that is fine. Once they have learned it, they should pronounce it more naturally.
- *Step 5: Provide the natural reward.* Give the child an opportunity to manipulate the tab as a natural reward.

Attention Seeking and Assistance Seeking

Many children with autism have no or few attention-seeking strategies in their repertoires and may not appear interested in seeking attention from others. However, these strategies are an important part of communication, and incorporating the PRT motivational strategies can make them rewarding for the child to use.

Attention-seeking strategies can be taught by prompting the child to say, "Look!" or "Watch me!" just before receiving a desired item or activity. For example, if the child enjoys swinging, you can prompt, "Look!" or "Look, Mommy!" just before pushing them. If the child is about to eat a popsicle on a hot day, you can gently hold the child's hand while prompting, "Look, I have a popsicle!" before the child eats it. Prompting attention-seeking phrases in motivational settings will provide the child with another language function and a social way of gaining attention.

Similarly, children may become frustrated when something is too difficult and may resort to inappropriate behaviors under these circumstances. Too often, teachers or other adults then prompt children to ask for help, but in the meantime, they have learned the cycle of 1) demonstrating behavior issues; 2) an adult approaching them and prompting them to ask for help; 3) asking for help and being rewarded with it. We want to break this cycle by making sure the request for help is the first "go-to," rather than beginning the process with behavior issues. For many children, requesting help requires a lot of practice before it becomes the fallback, so we initially start by setting up situations in which the child will not be able to be successful independently, and then prompt them to ask for help *before* they become frustrated. For example, we might screw a jar tightly with a treat inside and prompt the child to ask for help right away. Similarly, we might place a desired item a little out of reach and prompt the child to ask for help. By practicing this frequently, the child should become comfortable using the replacement behavior without the behavior issues. When a situation is set up and the child asks for help without needing a prompt, you have succeeded with enough practice. Be sure to confirm with other significant individuals in the child's life that the child is requesting help in various natural environments. If the child is not asking for help in other environments, spread the word that asking for help has been practiced and well established and needs to be prompted and practiced in those settings before the child becomes frustrated.

Social Interaction

Social interaction is often challenging for autistic individuals; however, those who are verbal indicate that they long for friends, significant others, and relationships. Too often, social areas are neglected, leaving autistic individuals without strategies for starting and maintaining relationships as adults. Because school settings contain a plethora of peers, it is essential that individualized education program goals include social goals. The question-asking described earlier helps the child engage in social verbal interactions with peers. The following are some additional goals that can be helpful in social interaction.

Play Initiation and Entering Play

Many children on the autism spectrum have an interest in peers but have not developed methods of play entry and initiation. Again, to increase the likelihood that play will be rewarding, these can be prompted during motivating activities. For example, if the child enjoys sliding down the slide, they can be encouraged to ask a peer to slide, with the natural reward being the opportunity to slide. Instead of an adult pushing the child on a swing, the child can be encouraged to ask a peer to push. If an ongoing activity is of interest to the autistic child, they can be encouraged to ask, "Can I play?" or preferred games and activities can be started with peers, and then the child can be prompted to ask to join.

Case Example: Ozzy

> Ozzy's parents reported that he enjoyed sifting sand at the seashore and could engage in this behavior repetitively for hours. However, at school, he only watched the other children play in the sandbox. Given that initiating play was a goal, his teacher asked his parents to send in some of his favorite sifting toys. Next, she prompted Ozzy to ask other children if they wanted to play in the sandbox. Once in the sandbox, the teacher prompted him to ask the other children if they wanted a sifter (sifters were very popular). Within a few days, Ozzy's peers were seeking him out at recess and were thrilled to engage with him. Importantly, Ozzy was learning play initiation, offering toys, and sharing—skills that are fundamental for making friends.

Case Example: Sara

> Sara was in elementary school when her parents noticed that she wandered the periphery of the schoolyard during all outdoor free play times while other children played in pairs or groups. To reverse this, Sara's parents selected a few of her favorite board games and taught her how to ask others if they wanted to play the game with her and how to explain the directions of the game. They sent these to school with her, and immediately after she was prompted to invite peers to join, a group of interested children came to the table. She often had to

explain the directions, giving her another opportunity to practice her communication.

Case Example: Gregory

Gregory was in kindergarten and spent recess periods alone, watching other children play. Suspecting that he longed to engage but was not skilled at entering play, his teacher prompted him to ask the other children if he could play with them. She remained in the area after the prompt to ensure that the children would include him once he asked. After a few weeks of prompting, Gregory easily asked the children if he could play and rarely was observed alone on the playground.

Turn-Taking

Learning to take turns is important for social interaction, but children often do not understand that turn-taking means that when they give up a toy for a peer's turn, it is not gone forever; they will get the toy back. This concept can be taught in the provider's office and demonstrated to parents. Say, "My turn," and gently take a toy, then give it back *immediately*. No delay. Try this several times, and when the child appears willing to give the item over for this brief period, add 1 second, then 2 seconds, then 3 seconds, and so on before giving it back. This way, the child will learn that the toy or desired item will be returned after a bit; "your turn" does not mean forever. You can also prompt the child to say, "Your turn" when giving the item over, which is a good phrase for many activities. If the child is not watching peers during their turn, it can be helpful for adults to teach them to watch the other child. Showing interest in others is important and can be started during these brief periods of turn-taking.

Case Example: Winston

Preschooler Winston spent hours lying on his side and repetitively opening and closing the small door of a playhouse. We included other children in this favorite activity by having them take turns opening and closing the door, labeling new vocabulary items such as "hinge" and "doorknob," and moving toy animals and people in and out of the playhouse door. Winston was also prompted to say, "Your turn" and "My turn" during these interactions.

Case Example: Jessie

> Jessie's favorite activity was playing with trains, and the school had a set that he functionally claimed as his own. He took the entire set to the corner and turned his back toward the other children. When classmates approached, he yelled at them, and they quickly retreated. To improve his socialization and turn-taking, we enforced the school's sharing rule that toys could only be played with in groups. He was taught to ask other children to play and to take turns putting the track pieces together and driving the trains on the track. With consistent teaching, he quickly learned not to exclude other children, not to yell when peers approached, and to enjoy the activity with peers.

Summary

Initiated communication, such as question-asking, leads to acquisition of additional linguistic and cognitive information and to social interactions. Without initiations, adults must create learning activities, and thus opportunities for learning and social interaction are unbalanced, with the autistic individual primarily responding to the communicative partner. Research shows that children who are taught initiations using the PRT motivational components have improved long-term outcomes (L.K. Koegel et al. 1999). A randomized clinical trial comparing a PRT intervention focused on initiations with a treatment-as-usual (TAU) group showed that when the intervention focused on initiations, greater gains were realized (Mohammadzaheri et al. 2022a). In addition, gains were shown in areas that were not specifically targeted, such as improvements in mean length of utterances (making longer sentences) and in overall composites of communicative skills (i.e., speech, syntax, initiation, coherence, stereotyped language, use of context, social relationship, rapport, and interests), as measured by the Children's Communication Checklist. These changes correlated with changes in electroencephalographic oscillations at several brain regions in the PRT group compared with the TAU group (Mohammadzaheri et al. 2022b).

For adolescents and adults who are verbal, questions can be practiced beforehand for more successful interactions (L.K. Koegel et al. 2021). Initiations can be taught in school, at the clinic, and through parent education (Popovic et al. 2020). The results of using a variety of questions and other initiations cannot be overemphasized as a pivotal area because they lead to a wide variety of gains in untargeted areas. Thus, initiations seem to be an especially important developmental area, and teaching these may produce added value in terms of short- and long-term benefits.

References

Koegel LK, Camarata SM, Valdez-Menchaca MC, et al: Setting generalization of question-asking and collateral language acquisition in children with autism. Am J Ment Retard 102:346–357, 1998 9475943

Koegel LK, Koegel RL, Shoshan Y, et al: Pivotal response intervention II: preliminary long-term outcome data. Res Pract Persons Severe Disabil 24(3):186–198, 1999

Koegel LK, Koegel RL, Green-Hopkins I, et al: Brief report: question-asking and collateral language acquisition in children with autism. J Autism Dev Disord 40(4):509–515, 2010 19936908

Koegel LK, Koplen Z, Koegel B, et al: Using a question bank intervention to improve socially initiated questions in adolescents and adults with autism. J Speech Lang Hear Res 64(4):1331–1339, 2021 33820435

Koegel LK, Ponder E, Nordlund KS, et al: Pivotal response treatment (PRT): research findings over 30 years, in Handbook of Applied Behavior Analysis Interventions for Autism: Integrating Research Into Practice. Cham, Switzerland, Springer International Publishing, 2022, pp 207–226

Koegel RL, Bradshaw JL, Ashbaugh K, et al: Improving question-asking initiations in young children with autism using pivotal response treatment. J Autism Dev Disord 44(4):816–827, 2014 24014174

Mohammadzaheri F, Koegel LK, Bakhshi E, et al: The effect of teaching initiations on the communication of children with autism spectrum disorder: a randomized clinical trial. J Autism Dev Disord 52(6):2598–2609 2022a 34296374

Mohammadzaheri F, Koegel LK, Soleymani Z, et al: Neural correlates of enhancing question asking and initiations in children with autism spectrum disorders: a randomized clinical trial. Soc Neurosci 17(2):181–192, 2022b 35296214

Popovic SC, Starr EM, Koegel LK: Teaching initiated question asking to children with autism spectrum disorder through a short-term parent-mediated program. J Autism Dev Disord 50(10):3728–3738, 2020 32112233

Wetherby AM: Ontogeny of communicative functions in autism. J Autism Dev Disord 16(3):295–316, 1986 3558289

4

Making Academics Fun and Meaningful

Academic Engagement

The level of participation in academics varies greatly across children, but parents of children on the autism spectrum often express concern that their child is making little progress on their individualized education program (IEP) goals, struggles with homework, and complains that they do not want to go to school. Engagement in academic activities is critical for success, and homework is an integral part of the educational process. Too often, children are rewarded for avoidance and escape-motivated behaviors that interfere with learning. This may occur inadvertently, such as when the child is removed from the classroom (sometimes brought to a "break room") or is released from an academic demand because they are exhibiting behaviors that function as ways to avoid academic tasks. This creates a vicious circle of low academic achievement and high levels of interfering behavior. Although many studies have shown that implementing reward systems can reduce these behaviors, a growing body of research suggests that the pivotal response treatment (PRT) motivational components can be incorporated into academics to produce high levels of academic engagement and interest, with generalization to other activities. For long-term success, developing an intrinsic desire to engage in academics will be far more enduring than completing work to gain a reward or to avoid punishment.

Overall health also may be an important factor related to success in school environments for children on the autism spectrum. Those who are a healthy weight, engage in physical activities, and have lower levels of screen time tend to be more engaged in school and more social (Garcia et al. 2023). Although these factors do not have a causal link with success in school, they are worth considering.

Homework

The implicit assumption is that homework should and can be completed independently, which leads to self-control and self-regulation. However, research suggests that parent involvement is important. For example, when students report that their parents play a supportive role in their homework, such as discussing homework, asking questions about it, offering help, providing encouragement, and answering questions, students complete more homework, put in more effort, and procrastinate less (Núñez et al. 2023). However, if the subject matter is difficult, parents may express negative feelings that transfer to their children and, consequently, decrease student motivation and enjoyment of the experience (Wu et al. 2022). Homework is a fundamental pedagogical activity used in schools worldwide, but the students who need homework most are often the least likely to engage in it. When children struggle with schoolwork or when their parents express stress while trying to help, this may undermine their success. For years, many aspects of homework have been widely debated, including its potential harm to mental and physical health, but for children on the autism spectrum, home and school collaboration can be helpful, if not essential.

Unfortunately, standard procedures relating to homework engagement and completion are lacking. They are best achieved when the home and school collaborate and coordinate effectively. Many teachers do not receive professional or pre-professional training on how to accomplish good home and school collaboration. Furthermore, because they teach large numbers of students, teachers frequently give insufficient feedback on homework assignments and on how parents can best support their children (Syla 2023).

The general literature on parent participation in homework suggests ensuring that the child is completing the homework independently and that the parents are not providing direct help that could hinder learning (e.g., giving correct answers, completing assignments). When homework becomes a struggle, parents too often resort to punitive measures rather than maintaining a positive attitude. Greater child-parent stress also can occur with low-achieving students, particularly as children grow and are expected to become increasingly independent with more challenging work. With education and training, parents can become more effective by making sure the homework environment is conducive to learning; helping with homework habits by setting rules, such as when and where the homework should be completed; providing proper supervision and support; and providing positive reinforcement for their child when rules are followed.

Improving Academic Engagement

Academics, both in school and as homework, can be a big challenge for children with autism because many demonstrate off-task behaviors to escape or avoid their work. However, psychiatrists and other health professionals can encourage parents and educators to incorporate PRT motivational components in order to improve academic engagement, which, in turn, will improve learning and behavior. Specific procedures can be suggested for teachers and parents to use at school and at home to make a difference in these children's academic progress.

Accumulating research shows that motivational components can improve academic engagement and homework completion. A study in which PRT was used (L.K. Koegel et al. 2010) showed that writing and math could be improved in elementary school students who initially exhibited various behaviors such as leaving the area, flopping on the floor, crying, yelling, kicking, spitting, melting down, and throwing task materials. Specifically, the PRT motivational components of choice, interspersal of maintenance tasks, and natural reinforcers were incorporated into the academic assignments to improve homework completion. Procedures included identifying child-preferred activities, which was accomplished through observation and parent report. These activities were incorporated into the homework assignments rather than provided as a reward, which provided an opportunity for a natural reinforcer rather than an arbitrary, unrelated reward. Choice was also implemented by allowing the students to choose where they wanted to complete their homework and the type of writing implement they wanted to use (e.g., pencil or marker). Additionally, some easier tasks were incorporated into the homework, interspersed with more difficult activities.

This study demonstrated that extrinsic rewards, even if preferred, did not improve the completion of homework problems. In fact, the periods in which off-task, interfering, and disruptive behaviors were exhibited before the child began the assignment steadily increased over time, often to 90%–100%. In contrast, when the PRT procedures were incorporated into the academics, the children's latency times decreased to negligible levels or were nonexistent, and interfering behaviors were at low levels or eliminated completely. Not surprisingly, work completion was high during the PRT academic sessions. The following vignettes are a few examples.

Case Example: Rob

Rob was fascinated by maps. His homework was to write paragraphs about a nonpreferred topic, but his teacher agreed to permit him to write about maps as long as he was learning how to create grammatically correct sentences and paragraphs that had an introduction, several detail sentences, and a conclusion. Rob was pleased to write about maps and quickly and competently completed his paragraphs without delaying the work or engaging in interfering behaviors.

Case Example: Gabe

Gabe enjoyed playing outside. However, when going outside was offered as a reward for writing sentences, he showed little interest and engaged in off-task behaviors, including laying down, yelling, spitting, and throwing objects. In contrast, when he was asked to write sentences about what he wanted to do outside, he quickly completed his sentences. Immediately after completing the sentences, he was provided with an opportunity to go outside and engage in those activities.

Case Example: Benito

Benito snacked on Cheerios after school, but when it came time to complete his addition and subtraction math homework, he exhibited behaviors such as meltdowns, kicking, and pinching. However, when he was provided with an opportunity to add and subtract the Cheerios, he came to the table immediately and participated willingly. Of course, he was able to eat the Cheerios once he completed the related math problems.

Case Example: Mylie

Mylie spent hours building with Legos but refused to engage in math activities. However, when Legos were used for the math calculations, such as adding up bricks of specific colors to calculate the number she would need to complete a figure, she enthusiastically completed advanced math calculations, with the natural reward of receiving the pieces to put together after the problems were completed.

Case Example: Jeffrey

Jeffrey was having a tough time learning how to read. By fourth grade, he had participated in numerous phonics programs that had not helped his reading. Frustrated, his mother began to incorporate PRT motivational components, selecting his favorite activities and items and teaching him to read their names before accessing them. Within just a few weeks, Jeffrey was able to read many different colors to get small M&M candies and had learned to read the words "pizza," "swing," "up," and "on." Once he began reading single words, his mother gradually prompted additional words until he could read complete sentences, such as "I want to turn on the television" and "Please give me one green and two blue candies." Furthermore, using these natural rewards provided an opportunity to assess his comprehension of the sentences.

While incorporating motivational components undoubtedly makes assignments more interesting, certain assignments may need to be completed in a particular way, and some teachers do not permit this type of task alteration. In such cases, PRT components can be used in a slightly different way. For example, children can be offered the choice of the writing implement they use, the color of the pen or marker, which problems they would like to complete in what order, what subject they would like to begin with or do next, and so on (Moes 1998). Offering these choices improves accuracy, engagement, and affect, and children engage in fewer interfering behaviors that take time away from learning.

Case Example: Brandon

Brandon was bright and fully included (meaning that he was placed full-time in general education courses) but engaged in off-task and avoidance behavior during homework. His parents struggled with getting him to begin assignments. Once they began providing him with a set of markers, letting him choose which color and type he wanted to use and asking him which assignment he wanted to do first, he showed improved cooperation and engagement in his homework.

Case Example: Courtney

Courtney struggled with school engagement. During a meeting, her parents suggested that the teacher implement opportunities for choice during academics because she appeared bored, and it was difficult to get her to begin her work. The teacher agreed and began searching for opportunities to include choice. For example, instead of providing only one writing topic, the teacher began offering three topics for her students to choose from. In addition, she provided different colors of paper for essays, so the students could choose among them. She also let her students sit anywhere in the classroom they chose while completing their independent assignments. All these choices resulted in increases in Courtney's engagement and correct responses and decreases in the latency time she took to start an assignment. Her parents also noted frequent positive comments about school. The teacher reported that she noticed improved enthusiasm and engagement in *all* her students, not just Courtney.

Case Example: Timmy

Timmy was placed in a special education classroom for students with autism. Several times a day, he escaped the classroom to run across the field and look at airplanes leaving from the nearby airport. An observing specialist noted that a large part of Timmy's curriculum included drill-type flash cards, presented by his one-to-one aide. His responses tended to be slow and infrequent, and he usually shook a pen throughout the lesson, spending more time looking at the pen than the flash cards. Given his interest in airplanes, we suggested that the curriculum be based around airplanes, including vocabulary, language, reading, math, and writing. As soon as the curriculum was restructured using his preferred theme of airplanes, Timmy began responding quickly and enthusiastically and no longer eloped from the classroom.

Research shows that teachers may need some training but can effectively use PRT variables in school, such as by providing students with choices both during and between activities, incorporating the students' interests and personalizing activities, interspersing easier with more difficult activities, using rewards directly related to the activity, and rewarding attempts. In randomized clinical trials with elementary school–aged children, significant improvements in engagement were seen when these motivational procedures were used (Stahmer et al. 2023). Most teachers report that they have not had training in using motivational strategies, but research shows that implementing PRT with fidelity results in improved student learning, therefore emphasizing the importance of teacher training in PRT (Stahmer et al. 2023). Alternatively, parents may request during an IEP or team meeting that PRT strategies be incorporated for their child. The more competent a teacher is at incorporating these strategies, the less off-task student behaviors will occur and the more students will learn, leading to more rapid progress toward student goals.

Summary

If a child with whom you work has low engagement with academic activities, an important question to ask is, "What procedures are being implemented to improve engagement?" Often, schools fall into a punishment-oriented routine of removing the child from the classroom or even sending the child home. These practices often are described as "a place for the child to calm down," "some downtime," or "quiet time," but because they are implemented in response to escape or avoidance behavior, they actually function as rewards because the child escapes the aversive or difficult academic activity. Although reward systems might be set up for students, these often do not create intrinsic motivation on the students' part to engage in the academic activity. As discussed, incorporating desired and preferred activities, themes, or topics into the curriculum can motivate students to engage in the curriculum. Even using restricted and repetitive behaviors in the curriculum can provide a highly rewarding activity for the student, and this does not appear to increase these behaviors at other times of the day (Baker et al. 1998; Brown and Stanton-Chapman 2015). Research shows that using PRT motivational components increases overall academic engagement, even when the student returns to less-preferred activities (Koegel et al. 2010). Thus, using an antecedent intervention, rather than a consequence-based intervention, leads to increased motivation, engagement, learning, positive student affect, and more accurate responses.

References

Baker MJ, Koegel RL, Koegel LK: Increasing the social behavior of young children with autism using their obsessive behaviors. J Assoc Pers Sev Handicaps 23(4):300–308, 1998

Brown TS, Stanton-Chapman T: Strategies for teaching children with autism who display or demonstrate circumscribed interests. Young Exceptional Children 18(4):31–40, 2015

Garcia JM, Hahs-Vaughn D, Shurack R: Health behaviors, psychosocial factors, and academic engagement in youth with autism spectrum disorder: a latent class analysis. Autism Res 16(1):143–153, 2023 36334019

Koegel LK, Singh AK, Koegel RL: Improving motivation for academics in children with autism. J Autism Dev Disord 40(9):1057–1066, 2010 20221791

Moes DR: Integrating choice-making opportunities within teacher-assigned academic tasks to facilitate the performance of children with autism. J Assoc Pers Sev Handicaps 23(4):319–328, 1998

Núñez JC, Freire C, Ferradás MDM, et al: Perceived parental involvement and student engagement with homework in secondary school: the mediating role of self-handicapping. Curr Psychol 42(6):4350–4361, 2023

Stahmer AC, Suhrheinrich J, Rieth SR, et al: A waitlist randomized implementation trial of classroom pivotal response teaching for students with autism. Focus Autism Other Dev Disabl 38(1):32–44, 2023 38605730

Syla LB: Perspectives of primary teachers, students, and parents on homework. Educational Research International 2023:7669108, 2023

Wu J, Barger MM, Oh DD, et al: Parents' daily involvement in children's math homework and activities during early elementary school. Child Dev 93(5):1347–1364, 2022 35435993

5

Addressing Interfering Behaviors

The Challenges of Interfering Behaviors

Interfering behaviors can disrupt family life, hinder learning, and hamper socialization. These behaviors include aggression, self-injurious behavior, property destruction, and, to a lesser extent, some restrictive and repetitive behaviors. Children diagnosed with autism are more likely to develop aggression than are those without autism.

Some reports suggest that more than half of autistic children will show aggression toward their parents, and about a third will show aggression toward other care providers (Mazurek et al. 2013). About 30% will demonstrate persistent aggression over time (Laverty et al. 2023). Communication challenges, sleep difficulties, sensory issues, social challenges, and gastrointestinal issues have all been reported to be associated with aggression (Mazurek et al. 2013). Self-injurious behavior and aggression sometimes co-occur with emotional dysregulation, including agitation, crying, screaming, whining, yelling, meltdowns, homicidal/suicidal statements, and so on (Northrup et al. 2022), which can be precursors to more intensive behaviors.

Why do interfering behaviors persist? For the most part, interfering behaviors are effective and efficient for the individual who is engaging in them. Most commonly, they are rewarded by tangibles (e.g., receiving the desired items or food after using undesired behavior), sensory reinforcement, attention, and/or escape or avoidance of a nonpreferred task or activity. Some children will demonstrate these behaviors some time prior to the actual aversive activity, which can make it difficult to see the pattern. Careful monitoring is important.

Understanding Interfering Behavior

First and foremost, assess whether motivational components are being incorporated into the teaching. It is unfair to provide poor teaching that results in interfering behaviors. Second, it is critical to understand the function of the interfering behavior and to address the cause if permanent change is to be realized. If motivational components clearly are being incorporated into the teaching and the individual continues to demonstrate interfering behaviors, an intervention program is warranted.

Over the years, the field has moved toward understanding the cause of interfering behaviors rather than punishing individuals for them because most of these behaviors have a communicative function. Understanding the function involves conducting a functional behavior assessment (FBA), which can be done in natural settings by observing the individual and hypothesizing the cause (Melanson and Fahmie 2023). Family members and others who know the child well can also provide information about the cause of the behavior. In some cases, verbal individuals can accurately report on their own functions (Dunlap et al. 1993). The purpose of an FBA is to determine the conditions and situations in which problem behaviors occur. This might be restricted to a specific academic task, an individual, or a setting. Once the function of a behavior is established, a support plan to replace interfering and inappropriate behaviors with functionally equivalent replacement behaviors (FERBs) is implemented.

Case Example: Ella

Ella's preschool teachers reported her repeated aggression with peers. Upon close observation, Ella lacked the verbal skills to request toys, so instead she forcefully grabbed them from peers. In addition, her challenges with social rules resulted in crowding and bumping into other children, which was perceived by her teachers as aggression.

Case Example: Tyler

During language arts class, Tyler exhibited whining and crying that escalated to property destruction when the teacher encouraged him to keep working on his assignments. During other times of the day, he exhibited no problem behaviors. The function of Tyler's behavior was in response to a class assignment that was too difficult for him, and he used the behavior to try to escape the assignment.

Case Example: Tommy

Tommy was bright, read a lot, and remembered almost everything he read. When an adult or another student made an inaccurate statement, such as "salty water boils quicker," he would begin to argue, yell, and then become aggressive toward the person who made the statement. The function of Tommy's behavior was to express disagreement with another person, especially when he was correct.

Case Example: Mona

Whenever Mona's mom talked on the telephone, Mona began whining. If her mother did not hang up quickly, Mona began pounding her head on the ground and hitting her head with a closed fist. This caused her mother great distress whenever the phone rang or she needed to make a phone call. The function of Mona's behavior was to get attention.

Decreasing Interfering Behaviors

The function of interfering behaviors can be assessed in several ways. A functional *analysis* differs from a functional *assessment* in that the environment is manipulated in order to understand the function of the behaviors. For example, a child may be given an easy assignment, then a hard one, then an easy one, alternating until a pattern appears. If the child demonstrates challenging behaviors every time a difficult assignment is given, the function is likely avoidance of difficult tasks. Most practitioners prefer to hypothesize about the function of a behavior using functional assessment (observation or informant methods); some consider it unethical to set up situations that are likely to elicit these behaviors. Simply observing in natural settings where these behaviors are reported to occur can yield invaluable information for developing a behavior plan.

Setting Events

Sometimes parents or teachers will report that their child or student is perfectly well-behaved most times but will occasionally have outbursts or meltdowns following an instruction with which the child typically complies. These are often determined to be related to *setting events*, or something in the past that predisposes the individual to respond differently than they generally would, usually with some sort of unwanted behavior. Setting events include prior events (internal or external) that increase the likelihood of an interfering behavior. These can be physiological variables, such as hunger, fatigue, pain, and illness. Other setting events may be unexpected occurrences that influence the course of the day, which for a child with autism can be something as seemingly simple as driving a different route to school, a fire alarm going off, or parents getting in an argument.

Case Example: Neil

Neil's paraprofessional was very punitive. Instead of encouraging Neil to behave well in class, she reminded him of past problematic episodes, which annoyed him. Whenever she reminded him of past events (e.g., "Don't act like you did yesterday in band. I don't want to see any tantrums. That isn't acceptable."), which happened often, he became agitated. Once agitated, he was more likely to have meltdowns after even a minor event in class.

Case Example: Brian

Brian enjoyed having his mother drive him to school each day. When road work was being done on their normal route, his mother had to take a detour. Following this detour, Brian exhibited numerous meltdowns when asked to complete his assignments that day at school.

Case Example: Sasha

Sasha had entered puberty and began menstruating. Once a month, cn the first day of her period, her discomfort caused her to exhibit aggression toward her teacher, particularly during academics. Although she generally engaged willingly in academics, this aggression was a monthly occurrence.

Case Example: Joseph

Joseph was generally well-behaved until his mother had a second child. The new child awoke several times during the night, which also caused Joseph to wake up. His fatigue caused him to have regular meltdowns at school.

Again, current strategies to address these behaviors involve examining the function of the behavior and teaching FERBs. If setting events are an issue, the demands can be decreased, and the influential variable can be addressed. For example, if the child is engaging in meltdowns because they are hungry, more frequent snacks can be provided. If the young adult has menstrual cramps, heating pads and aspirin can be helpful. One cautionary note: although, on occasion, physiological variables are the cause of behavior issues, it is important to attempt to fully understand the function of interfering behaviors rather than simply dismissing them as physiological.

As mentioned, most interfering behaviors are communicative, and parents need to understand that these behaviors are likely to return if the child does not learn an appropriate way to express the communicative function of the interfering behavior. The behaviors can worsen over time and become more harmful as the individual grows; therefore, attending to them at the earliest point in time is warranted.

When meeting with families who report interfering behaviors, it is helpful for the psychiatrist or provider to understand the most common functions of these behaviors (Table 5.1). Although the functions of most interfering behaviors can be determined, some have multiple functions or are used more generally.

Interfering behaviors can persist over time because they are both efficient and effective. If a child hits classmates when they attempt to play with his favorite toys, the classmates will stay away, leaving him with all the toys. If a child screams to get a cookie before dinner, a parent may give her the cookie to stop the screaming. A child who engages

---

Table 5.1 Common functions of interfering behaviors

Escape	Many autistic children engage in interfering behaviors in an attempt to avoid an undesired task or activity. For example, they may swipe classroom materials off the table if they do not enjoy the subject or an assignment is too difficult. For some children, sensory issues, such as loud noises or a fire alarm at school, may cause problem behavior.
Avoidance	Some children will begin engaging in interfering behaviors before an activity starts. For example, one student complained of feeling sick every day just before math class. Another engaged in a meltdown whenever a particular and/or demanding provider arrived at his home.
Attention	Many autistic children do not engage in attention-seeking behavior because they are less inclined to interact socially. However, occasionally a child will engage in behaviors when a parent is on the phone or talking to another adult. Some children will repeatedly ask for items or ask the same question over and over to maintain an adult's attention. We have even seen children hit or push other children when they want to play but do not have a way to appropriately communicate this desire.
Tangible (grabbing objects)	A child who lacks communication may grab items or display other behaviors (e.g., crying, screaming) if they are not provided with immediate access to a desired item or activity.
Transition or perseveration of sameness	Transitions are challenging for many people, especially when they are moving from a preferred to a less or nonpreferred activity. Some children will engage in interfering behavior at most transitions, regardless of whether they are preferred or not. Similarly, some autistic children will react when there is a change in routine, when the order of a group of toys they have lined up is altered, or when the furniture is changed.
Excitement	Rarely, autistic children will show a behavior, usually self-injury, when excited. For example, one child ran in circles while biting his wrist when he was excited.

Table 5.1 Common functions of interfering behaviors *(continued)*

Restricted and repetitive behavior (RRB)	On rare occasions a child will engage in an RRB that is not the result of external events and can sometimes evolve into self-injury. For example, one child picked at his skin repetitively until it bled, which created scabs that he further picked. These RRBs have no communicative function and therefore require a different strategy for addressing. They often occur when the child is alone. For example, one child repeatedly bit himself on the wrist while playing outside on his swing set when no others were present.

---

in a meltdown rather than starting their classwork may be taken to a quiet room to "calm down," therefore successfully avoiding the academic task. In all these instances, the behavior is working and thus will likely be used again in the future.

Treatment: Functionally Equivalent Replacement Behaviors

The first step in addressing interfering behaviors is to figure out the function or, in some cases, functions of the behavior. Once you have hypothesized a function—through observation or by interviewing the individual or others who interact with them—you will need to develop a replacement behavior that serves the same function as the behavior you want to eliminate. As mentioned earlier, these are referred to as *functionally equivalent replacement behaviors,* or FERBs. There are a few general rules when developing and teaching a replacement behavior:

- **Keep everyone safe.** Do not worry about implementing an intervention during a crisis situation. Make sure that everyone is safe, including the child engaging in the behavior. You can focus on developing an intervention program once the event has passed and everyone is calm.
- **Make it easy.** Interfering behaviors are efficient and effective, so the replacement behavior should be just as easy to use in the moment. For example, if the individual is nonverbal and engages in aggression when an activity is too long, teaching them to sign

"I want break" (three signs) may be too laborious, and they will likely resort to the easier and equally effective behavior of aggression. Teaching one sign—that is, "break"—is more useful. Similarly, if a child gets upset every time another child takes a toy, teaching them to say "Please give me back my toy" may be too difficult. Teaching "mine" serves the same function and is much easier. Later, once the replacement behavior is well established, longer utterances can be prompted.

- **Practice, practice, practice.** A common mistake when teaching replacement behaviors is prompting the FERB only after an interfering behavior occurs. The risk here is that the individual may learn a pattern of behaviors: "First I hit, then the teacher comes over and prompts me to say 'mine,' then I say 'mine' and get the toy back." In this scenario, the subsequent steps only occur after the initial inappropriate behavior and end with a rewarding consequence, thus reinforcing the chain of behaviors. Situations should be set up for practice throughout the day when the individual is not frustrated, irritated, or engaging in an interfering behavior. For example, Baron became upset whenever he could not get a toy to work properly, at which point he would hurl the toy across the room. This often resulted in property damage and injury to another child. His teachers intervened by identifying the toys that might frustrate him and then prompting him to say "help," at which time they offered help. With frequent practice, he rapidly learned that "help" was effective in getting the toy working, and this became his preferred communication.

- **Make problem behaviors ineffective.** When teaching the replacement behavior, it is preferable to make the interfering behaviors ineffective whenever possible. In some situations, the interfering behavior can be ignored. If the FERB has been practiced enough, the individual is likely to search for a response that will work, and that will likely be the FERB. For example, Dane enjoyed his mother's attention. Although most of the time he could get it readily, when she was engaged in conversation with another person, on the phone, or working, he would poke her, nudge her, and whine, behaviors that escalated if she did not quickly provide attention. In place of this behavior, he was taught to say "Excuse me," at which time she immediately gave him her attention. She then ignored him whenever he engaged in one of the interfering behaviors. Similarly, when Jess wanted a toy or food item, she aggressively grabbed it, which upset the other children. Because Jess was verbal, she was taught to say "Cracker, please" or "Car, please." Her teachers made sure she was not able to obtain the items when she tried to grab them, and Jess quickly learned that using the FERB was effective and that aggressively grabbing was not.

- **Teach tolerating a delay.** Children need to learn patience and that not everything happens immediately. This concept may be more difficult for individuals on the autism spectrum who have communication challenges. Once an individual has learned to use a FERB, it is important to gradually and systematically teach them to tolerate a delay. At first, they should be rewarded immediately upon using a replacement behavior. However, in real life it is not always practical to follow through immediately, and this may necessitate setting up times to practice tolerating a delay. Dane, for example—who sought his mother's attention when she was unavailable—quickly learned that he could get her attention by saying "Excuse me." Our support staff made frequent calls to Dane's mom so that she could abruptly end the call when he used the appropriate replacement behavior. However, once he was using the newly learned replacement behavior, his mother began putting up her finger and waiting 1 second before giving him attention. Gradually, she increased the delay to 2 seconds, 3, 4, 5, 10, 20, and so on. By doing this gradually and systematically, she taught Dane to tolerate the wait time and that the desired reward would come eventually, not immediately.

- **Use pivotal response treatment (PRT) points when teaching FERBs.** When setting up situations to practice FERBs, make sure they are motivational. For example, if a child displays interfering behaviors whenever they need help, place a favorite treat or toy in a plastic jar with the lid screwed on a bit too tightly for the child. Immediately, the replacement behavior of saying "Help" or "Please help" can be prompted. The child should then receive the desired item as a reward for using the FERB. If children associate positive outcomes with using FERBs, they will be more likely to use them in future situations.

Although several programs are effective at reducing interfering behaviors, if children have not learned an appropriate way to communicate their wants, needs, and feelings, the interfering behaviors are likely to return. For this reason, it is critical to determine the function or functions of a behavior and to work on teaching replacement behaviors.

However, the FERB often takes a bit of time to teach, so complement-
ing this program with another may be helpful for quickly reducing the
interfering behavior while simultaneously teaching the replacement.
The following are some programs that can be helpful in reducing interfering behaviors.

Antecedent Strategies

Prevention is always desired when behaviors exist that may cause
injuries, destroy property, or disrupt an ongoing activity. A number of
strategies can be put in place beforehand that lower the probability of
behaviors occurring.

Predictability

Providing a schedule so that daily activities are expected is helpful
across the age span, especially if transitions are difficult. The schedule
can be shown to the individual in the morning and throughout the day.
Similarly, a countdown or timer is helpful for transitions, particularly if
the individual is moving from a desired to a less desired activity.

Ecological Manipulations

The environment can be changed to reduce interfering behaviors in
some cases. An example might be changing a seating arrangement. One
child sat near her infant sibling at the dinner table and was aggressive
every time the infant banged her spoon on the table. Placing her more
than an arm's length away from the infant gave the parents time to stop
the banging before the child's aggression occurred. Sometimes it may
help to place a child near a preferred and competent peer who can offer
support when the child is frustrated in school. Some children have better behavior with preferential seating toward the front of the classroom,
others toward the back, and others when sandwiched between classmates. One child we worked with in school had increases in behavior
when he was facing the window. Preferential seating should be discussed as an antecedent option. Furthermore, it is common for autistic
individuals to be bullied, which can result in problematic behaviors;
thus, identifying and educating the bully can be effective. For some,
small things that cause sensory issues, such as certain fabrics that are
uncomfortable, clothing tags, or loud noises, can lead to behaviors, and
these often can be avoided beforehand. Changing the environment,
within reason, can be helpful in decreasing behaviors.

Priming

Another antecedent strategy is previewing materials before they are presented in class (L.K. Koegel et al. 2003). Some individuals engage in interfering behaviors when the assignment is difficult or when attempting to avoid an upcoming activity. *Priming* simply involves previewing an activity before it is presented in class or in the natural environment. Priming is often provided in the home setting and implemented in a fun and non-demanding manner. The point is to familiarize the child with the work, not to exhaust the material. If parents are unavailable, a school staff member can prime the child. Priming can be added to the child's individualized education program to ensure home and school coordination and implementation. We have successfully implemented priming with all academic subjects, story time, field trips, team sports, games, and so on.

Social Stories

Social stories are similar to priming in that social situations and the appropriate behaviors for those situations are explained to the child beforehand (Gray et al. 2002). Pictures are often used, and each step is explained to the child along with the expected behaviors. Reviews have stressed that the social stories should be simple and read immediately before the targeted situation. Implementation should include functional assessment to inform the intervention. Frequent check-ins for comprehension are also advised. Social stories seem to be most effective with elementary school–aged children who are included in regular education and have higher levels of communication (Kokina and Kern 2010).

Consequence-Based Interventions

Reward Systems

Rewarding children for desired behaviors can improve behavior, self-esteem, and peer acceptance. When children are demonstrating interfering behavior, good behaviors may go unnoticed and unrewarded. As a psychiatrist or provider, you may want to ask your patient how good behavior is being rewarded. Many teachers have a "demerit" system, wherein a specific number of disruptive behaviors results in a larger consequence, such as being sent to the principal's office, removed from the classroom, or given after-school detention. These types of punishments could be easily replaced with reward systems with the same, if not better, outcomes. Implementing a systematic reward system wherein good behavior is acknowledged and rewarded can make a difference. Reward systems can range from praise or direct rewards to tokens that can be accumulated and exchanged later for a desired item or activity. The reward must be self-chosen, particularly for autistic individuals. Furthermore, reward systems need to start with a short enough duration or number of responses to be worthwhile. The individual needs to know exactly what they are working toward and what they are required to do to reach that goal. Expectations should be clearly defined for them, and their understanding of these expectations must be confirmed. Sometimes behavior contracts are written for the individual to sign after agreeing to the expectations, particularly for verbal individuals (Hawkins et al. 2011). "First-then" instructions (e.g., "First reading, then free play") are generally provided when implementing a reward system.

Reward systems do not preclude random rewards for good behavior that is caught in the moment but are set up to be consistent and systematic. Additionally, reward systems need to be faded over time to more closely approximate the natural environment. For some children, fading may need to occur slowly; fading too quickly may result in increases in unwanted behavior. Behaviors also may not generalize to other settings, so coordination of reward systems across settings may be necessary.

Self-Management

Self-management programs have the advantage of helping individuals learn to evaluate their own behavior and lend themselves to more rapid fading of a support person. Chapter 6, "Self-Control Through Self-Management," describes such programs in detail; they can be put in place to quickly reduce unwanted behaviors while focusing on teaching FERBs. In addition to being used in combination with other programs, self-management programs have also been used to record the use of FERBs or other target behaviors in natural environments (L.K. Koegel et al. 1992).

Video Modeling

With the advent of small, portable video recorders, video modeling has become a more practical tool for behavior management. Although observational learning in natural settings may be challenging for individuals on the autism spectrum, the use of video modeling has proven to be effective and sometimes can be more effective than in vivo modeling (Charlop-Christy et al. 2000). Video modeling can be implemented by recording the individual (video self-modeling) or by showing the individual video examples of another person. When using video modeling, similarity to the target individual is recommended, as is the use of multiple examples to promote generalization. The general steps include showing the individual short video clips and discussing the desired behaviors shown. Some studies have also sandwiched examples of behaviors that "need improvement" between examples of the desired behaviors. This provides an opportunity for the individual to discuss different appropriate behaviors that could be used in that situation (Tagavi et al. 2021). Video modeling programs have targeted a variety of areas, including socialization, on-task behavior, function, self-help, and academics (Bellini and Akullian 2007).

Summary

Again, most interfering behaviors serve a communicative function. Aggression and property destruction are behaviors commonly used to escape a task or activity and to access tangibles. Self-injurious behavior is frequently demonstrated to escape task demands or for automatic reinforcement, and stereotypic behavior is most often exhibited for automatic reinforcement (Healy et al. 2013). Determining the function of the behavior and teaching replacement behaviors are critical for the long-lasting elimination of unwanted behaviors. Additionally, a multicomponent intervention program is recommended for addressing interfering behaviors. Antecedent interventions that prevent or reduce the likelihood of interfering behaviors occurring are essential, and regular reminders of expected behaviors are important. Once a program is implemented, constant monitoring and evaluation should occur because different things work better for different people. When a patient is engaging in interfering behaviors, observe how these behaviors are being dealt with at present; common school-based strategies, such as removing a student from the classroom, sending them to the office, and/or suspending them, often reward these escape- and avoidance-motivated behaviors. The same can be the case at home, where some parents report feeling as though they are "walking on eggshells" trying to avoid significant behaviors. Psychiatrists and other providers can alert parents to common oversights that maintain these behaviors in school, home, and community settings.

Psychiatrists and providers also can make recommendations of positive, evidence-based approaches to improve areas correlated with behavior and mental health issues, such as the eating and sleeping challenges frequently experienced by autistic individuals. Addressing these areas and decreasing interfering behaviors can help improve the quality of life. Fortunately, punishment that was used in the past to decrease these behaviors is no longer necessary (Carr et al. 2002) because ample positive behavior support strategies are available, some of which have been described in this chapter. Finally, good teaching using the PRT components can be an antidote to interfering behaviors and can eliminate the need for specialized programming because these behaviors become reduced or absent once motivational components are incorporated into the curriculum (L.K. Koegel et al. 2010; R.L. Koegel et al. 1992; Mohammadzaheri et al. 2015).

References

Bellini S, Akullian J: A meta-analysis of video modeling and video self-modeling interventions for children and adolescents with autism spectrum disorders. Except Child 73(3):264–287, 2007

Carr EG, Dunlap G, Horner RH, et al: Positive behavior support: evolution of an applied science. J Posit Behav Interv 4(1):4–16, 2002

Charlop-Christy MH, Le L, Freeman KA: A comparison of video modeling with in vivo modeling for teaching children with autism. J Autism Dev Disord 30(6):537–552, 2000 11261466

Dunlap G, Kern L, Deperczel M, et al: Functional analysis of classroom variables for students with emotional and behavioral disorders. Behav Disord 18(4):275–291, 1993

Gray C, White AL, McAndrew S: My Social Stories Book. Philadelphia, PA, Jessica Kingsley Publishers, 2002

Hawkins E, Kingsdorf S, Charnock J, et al: Using behaviour contracts to decrease antisocial behaviour in four boys with an autistic spectrum disorder at home and at school. Br J Spec Educ 38(4):201–208, 2011

Healy O, Brett D, Leader G: A comparison of experimental functional analysis and the Questions About Behavioral Function (QABF) in the assessment of challenging behavior of individuals with autism. Res Autism Spectr Disord 7(1):66–81, 2013

Koegel LK, Koegel RL, Hurley C, et al: Improving social skills and disruptive behavior in children with autism through self-management. J Appl Behav Anal 25(2):341–353, 1992 1634427

Koegel LK, Koegel RL, Frea W, et al: Priming as a method of coordinating educational services for students with autism. Lang Speech Hear Serv Sch 34(3):228–235, 2003 27764324

Koegel LK, Singh AK, Koegel RL: Improving motivation for academics in children with autism. J Autism Dev Disord 40(9):1057–1066, 2010 20221791

Koegel RL, Koegel LK, Surratt A: Language intervention and disruptive behavior in preschool children with autism. J Autism Dev Disord 22(2):141–153, 1992 1378049

Kokina A, Kern L: Social story interventions for students with autism spectrum disorders: a meta-analysis. J Autism Dev Disord 40(7):812–826, 2010 20054628

Laverty C, Agar G, Sinclair-Burton L, et al: The 10-year trajectory of aggressive behaviours in autistic individuals. J Intellect Disabil Res 67(4):295–309, 2023 36654499

Mazurek MO, Kanne SM, Wodka EL: Physical aggression in children and adolescents with autism spectrum disorders. Res Autism Spectr Disord 7(3):455–465, 2013

Melanson IJ, Fahmie TA: Functional analysis of problem behavior: a 40-year review. J Appl Behav Anal 56(2):262–281, 2023 36892835

Mohammadzaheri F, Koegel LK, Rezaei M, et al: A randomized clinical trial comparison between pivotal response treatment (PRT) and adult-driven applied behavior analysis (ABA) intervention on disruptive behaviors in public school children with autism. J Autism Dev Disord 45(9):2899–2907, 2015 25953148

Northrup JB, Goodwin MS, Peura CB, et al: Mapping the time course of overt emotion dysregulation, self-injurious behavior, and aggression in psychiatrically hospitalized autistic youth: a naturalistic study. Autism Res 15(10):1855–1867, 2022

Tagavi D, Koegel L, Koegel R, et al: Improving conversational fluidity in young adults with autism spectrum disorder using a video-feedback intervention. J Posit Behav Interv 23(4):245–256, 2021

6

Self-Control Through Self-Management

Creating Independence

Although the motivational strategies in pivotal response treatment (PRT) can make a huge difference in learning and behavior, self-control and self-regulation are also pivotal for development. At a certain point, children, adolescents, and adults need to take control of their own behaviors. Nonautistic children often acquire self-management and self-control without needing a specialized program. However, many autistic individuals may benefit from a systematic program designed to meet this need. Self-management can be programmed into natural settings and can address a wide range of behaviors. Self-management procedures are used to teach individuals to identify the presence or absence of a behavior, self-record the presence or absence of that behavior, and, in some cases, self-administer a reward for engaging—or *not* engaging—in the behavior. Becoming aware of and monitoring one's own behaviors greatly reduces the need for an interventionist by shifting the responsibility to the individual (Harrower and Dunlap 2001).

This can be especially important for older elementary school–aged children and beyond, who may be stigmatized by having an adult or provider present in everyday settings.

Over time, self-management programs can be created to initiate behavior changes that ultimately will be reinforced by consequences occurring naturally in the learners' everyday environments. For example, an adolescent with social challenges who learns to self-record responses to peers during social conversations may initially turn in points for desired rewards but eventually might receive a great deal of positive social attention from peers. Thus, the behavior is maintained by these rewarding interactions. For most behaviors, learners are gradually and systematically weaned from the initial external rewards until the target behavior is maintained by the natural environmental reinforcers. In many cases, we see desired behaviors increase without the learner needing to record every response, but in some cases, fading is more challenging and some sort of system needs to remain in place.

Self-management can be very effective for addressing interfering behaviors but should not be considered a replacement for good teaching. Teachers often do not individualize their curriculum for children on the autism spectrum (which, incidentally, should be done for all children), implement drill-like and monotonous exercises, or have a slow and boring delivery. In such cases, improving the delivery of the curriculum with PRT motivational strategies is a most desirable first step (as discussed in Chapter 4, "Making Academics Fun and Meaningful"). Furthermore, although self-management can work quickly, individuals must be taught a replacement behavior for aggression, self-injury, property destruction, and other interfering behaviors (as discussed in Chapter 5, "Addressing Interfering Behaviors"). Self-management may decrease or even eliminate these behaviors, but for it to make lasting gains and ensure communicative competence, the function of the behavior should always be considered; this should be assessed and addressed before or while a self-management program is being implemented.

Many reviews have shown that self-management is evidence-based and effective for increasing or decreasing behaviors in preschoolers, elementary school–aged children, adolescents, and adults on the autism spectrum. Self-management programs have been used to improve areas related to socialization, including social responsiveness to others (L.K. Koegel et al. 1992), question-asking (Palmen et al. 2008), social initiations (Deitchman et al. 2010), pragmatic areas (L.K. Koegel et al. 2014), social conversation (Newman et al. 1996), and sharing (Reinecke et al. 1999). In addition, appropriate play has been taught to children through self-management (Stahmer and Schreibman 1992).

Studies have also documented the effectiveness of self-management for improving academics, including overall engagement (Cihak et al. 2010), engagement in inclusive settings (Hart and Whalon 2008), on-task behavior, and homework completion (with parents implementing the program) (Simmons et al. 2022). Studies have shown that self-management can be a useful tool for reducing interfering repetitive and restricted behaviors in inclusive classroom settings (R.L. Koegel and Koegel 1990), as well as decreasing challenging behaviors such as aggression, property destruction, and tantrums (Carr 2016). In addition, self-management programs have been used in work settings to target task completion (Ganz and Sigafoos 2005) and improve daily living skills (Newman et al. 1995).

As can be noted from the large number and variety of studies, self-management is a flexible procedure that can easily be adapted to individuals of various age ranges, different target areas, and a large array of settings and can be used in combination with the PRT motivational strategies.

General Self-Management Steps

A self-management program can be set up during an office visit, although support in the natural setting where it is expected to occur may be necessary. Teaching self-management varies somewhat across studies, but the basic procedures involve the following steps.

Step 1A: Define and Measure the Target Behavior

First, begin by defining and measuring the target behavior in the settings where improvement is desired. A specific and detailed definition is important so that progress can be measured and the individual using self-management understands what is expected. Always think about what the behavior is and what you would like to see in that situation. Defining the desired behavior is important because when we implement self-management systems, we like to focus on the positive. Rather than having a child self-manage "no hitting or slapping," we might phrase this as "having calm, quiet hands" or "being nice to friends." In many cases, a parent or individual will report a behavior of concern before the office visit, which is helpful for pre-planning. The behavior must be very clearly explained to ensure that the individual understands what is expected.

- Example of a poorly defined target behavior: good behavior in class.
- Example of a well-defined target behavior: stay in seat, actively work on academic tasks assigned by the teacher, raise hand (instead of calling out).

After defining the target behavior(s) very specifically, measure the behavior in the natural setting where the self-management will take place. Sometimes this can be assessed in an office, but it is helpful to ask parents if the behavior is similar in natural settings. This will assist in determining an appropriate starting point for self-management and will serve as a baseline comparison for assessing whether the program is effective or needs adjustment. It also will help with communication among everyone involvedAfter defining the target behavior(s) very specifically, measure the behavior in the natural setting where the self-management will take place. Sometimes this can be assessed in an office, but it is helpful to ask parents if the behavior is similar in natural settings. This will assist in determining an appropriate starting point for self-management and will serve as a baseline comparison for assessing whether the program is effective or needs adjustment. It also will help with communication among everyone involved.

Step 1B: Identify Rewards

Next, identify a reward for the individual to earn once they reach the predetermined number of points. This is best accomplished by simply asking the individual what they would like to earn. Parents can sometimes be helpful with this and can bring rewards to the office visit. What is rewarding varies greatly across individuals, and sometimes a reward that was chosen in the past is no longer motivating, so it is helpful to consider the individual's interests and have a variety of rewards available. One young adult who was majoring in physics chose to give his support providers physics lessons as a reward when he earned a specific number of points. Children's choices range from stickers or small toys to earning time to play a video game or going out for pizza. Making sure the rewards are desirable and powerful is important. Generally, we start with smaller rewards and work up to larger ones as the individual becomes more independent.

Step 2: Develop a Monitoring System

If the desired behavior can be measured in numbers, such as each time the person raises their hand or answers a question, a tally system can be used. Tallies can be marked on a simple wrist counter (golf counters are great and inexpensive), on non-wrist counters (I always keep a variety of counters in my office and give the individual a choice of which they prefer), or even on a piece of paper. For continuous behaviors that will be measured in time intervals, such as staying in their seat or reading quietly during silent reading time, a timer on a watch or phone can be used, along with a sheet of paper with a box representing each interval.

During the self-management program, the individual will record occurrences (or intervals) of the desired behavior, so it is important to also choose a monitoring system that is easy to use and appropriate for the context.

Case Example: Abel

Abel responded to questions about half of the time. To improve his responsiveness, he was given a wrist counter that he wore throughout the day.

Case Example: Darren

Darren's teacher complained that he constantly called out answers and did not raise his hand as expected in her classroom, despite continual reminders. To reverse this pattern, a timer was placed on his desk, and he was given a checklist. Using this system, he tallied every interval during which he raised his hand to answer without calling out.

Case Example: Jonathan

The time between when Jonathan was asked to do his homework and when he started his homework varied from 10 to 15 minutes. His mother constantly reminded him to do his homework, using phrases such as "Let's do your homework," "It's time to get your homework done," and "Sit down now and start your homework." She reminded him approximately three times per minute. During this time, Jonathan protested (e.g., "I don't want to"), made off-task responses (e.g., "Can I have a snack? I'm so hungry"), and engaged in off-task behaviors, such as lying on the floor, whining, and refusing to go to the table. Once Jonathan got to the table, he engaged in homework for 2–3 minutes before leaving the area.

Desired behaviors: Come to the table the first time you are asked, start your homework right away, and keep working on it until the timer rings.

Data were collected on 1) how many reminders were needed; 2) how long it took Jonathan to begin his homework; and 3) how long he engaged in homework. Because the time he initially spent doing homework before starting the self-management program was 2–3 minutes, the first interval goal was 1 minute, with no delay in starting, to ensure he would be successful, and then the goal was quickly increased by 1-minute intervals until he reached 15 minutes.

Case Example: Emily

Emily responded to others' questions slightly more than 40% of the time. With her mother, she responded to an average of 6 out of every 10 questions. With her peers, she responded to 3 out of every 10 questions. With her teacher, she responded to 5 out of every 10 questions.

Desired behavior: Answer questions every time people ask.

Emily began recording each response on a wrist counter. Because she ranged from 40% to 60% responsiveness, we began rewarding her after each response on her wrist counter (then rapidly increased the rewards to every 2 answers, every 3, every 4, and so on until she was responding to 20 consecutive questions before she received a reward, which is described in the fading step below).

Once you have collected information on how often the behavior occurs, obtained a self-monitoring sheet or device, and set a target goal, you can begin teaching the individual to self-manage their own behavior.

Step 3: Teach Discrimination

During this third step, the individual must convey their understanding of what will be expected. It is helpful to begin with the contrast between the target behavior and other behaviors. Start by explaining the expectations (e.g., "We're going to work on staying focused so you can get your homework finished quickly"), then demonstrate some examples of behaviors seen or reported at baseline, along with the target behavior(s). After each demonstration, ask the child to determine whether you are engaging in the target behavior (e.g., "staying focused") or not. For example, I might lean back in my chair and look around, then ask the student if that is "staying focused." Next, I sit up straight and engage in some work, then ask the student if that is "staying focused." This is repeated with each behavior (or as many as possible) observed during step 1 until the individual can accurately discriminate the presence or absence of the target behavior. Once the individual clearly understands what is expected and is correctly identifying the target behavior versus other behaviors, they can be taught how to engage in the desired behaviors and how to self-record when they are demonstrated.

Case Example: Marcus

> Marcus, an elementary school student, frequently left his desk and made loud noises that interfered with his own work and the work of others. His team decided that a self-management program for "sitting nicely" should be implemented. When teaching Marcus to discriminate between the presence and absence of the target behavior (i.e., sitting nicely), his interventionist asked Marcus, "Is this sitting nicely?" while getting out of the seat and then asked, "Is this sitting nicely?" while sitting in the seat. Similarly, for sitting quietly without making interfering repetitive noises, the adult made noises and then asked Marcus, "Is this quiet sitting?" or modeled sitting quietly and asked, "Is this quiet sitting?"

After the child correctly answers the question "Is this [target behavior]?" regarding the absence or presence of the target behavior(s), they should immediately be given feedback, a high five, praise, or a small reward. When the child is incorrect, rather than being reprimanded, they can be asked to "try again." This can be practiced until the child can identify both the presence and the absence of the target behavior(s) and you are sure they have a good understanding of that behavior. Generally, when self-management is ineffective, it is because the individual does not have a clear understanding of the appropriate behavior.

Once the individual understands the expectations, they are taught how to record the desired behavior. The important thing to remember is that the adults will no longer immediately provide feedback regarding the target behavior; at this point, the individual will evaluate themselves as to whether they used the behavior. Parents and professionals sometimes need some training with this because their first instinct is to give feedback right away (e.g., "good job" or "not quite"). The individual should be given the chance to reflect on their own behavior rather than relying on an outside source for feedback.

Step 4: Teach Engagement and Recording

Now it is time to teach the individual to actively self-manage the target behavior. Teaching engagement and recording of the target behavior is usually done in a one-on-one setting. I generally start this program during office visits so the parents have a good idea of how to implement the program and can see the dramatic and rapid improvements that can ensue. Once the process is learned, it can easily be programmed to occur in natural settings.

In this fourth step, explain to the individual that when they engage in the target behavior, they can mark the occurrence on the recording device and then turn in their "points" for rewards. If the individual will be self-managing behavior for a specific time interval, the end of the interval must be specified. The timer function on the phone can be used; the individual can be taught to press the cancel button to stop the timer and the start button to begin the next interval. Some watches and phones have repeat chronograph alarm functions, so the individual would not have to manually stop and restart the alarm. Vibrating watches can also be used so that no alarm sounds. As the intervals are lengthened, it is practical to strive to increase the time periods to coincide with naturally occurring breaks during the day (e.g., the end of each class period or recess if self-management is being used in school) for self-recording.

Next, review the rewards and ask the individual what they would like to earn. For some children, it is motivating to have the rewards in sight so they can be reminded of what they are working toward. At this point, you can determine the number of points or successfully completed intervals that need to be earned to receive the reward.

Moving onward, explain that after the target behavior is used, the individual can check the counter or box. If you are using an interval system, be sure to start with an interval that is shorter than the shortest average interval at baseline. For example, if the interfering behavior was noted to occur once per minute, you may want to start with 15 or 30 seconds for the target behavior. In some instances, the starting interval may be 3–5 seconds. If you are counting discrete successful behaviors using a wrist counter, counting device, or sheet of paper, show the individual how to engage in the behavior (e.g., by asking a question) and how to record it. Then, prompt them to engage in the behavior and to self-record immediately afterward. If these steps (engaging in the target behavior and recording it) are performed correctly, praise the individual and prompt again. If either the target behavior or the recording does not occur, remind the individual and try again.

Case Example: Nathan

> Nathan was a kindergarten student on the autism spectrum who repeatedly called out answers in class without first raising his hand. He was bright and did this constantly, which the teacher reported to be "extremely annoying and unfair to the other students." To help him learn to raise his hand and not call out, Nathan was taken through the self-management steps, then given a counter to use in class. Initially, this process was monitored by the school psychologist, who reported that it was not working as intended; Nathan frequently called out and then immediately covered his mouth with his hands, suggesting that he realized he had engaged in the behavior that was being addressed. The school psychologist allowed him to give himself a point because, according to her, "he tried." Once we adjusted the program so that Nathan gave himself points only when he raised his hand and did not call out and not when he caught himself after calling out, his calling out decreased to negligible levels.

Again, ensuring that the expectations are completely clear is critical to success.

Step 5: Reward the Individual

Initially, self-management programs are introduced to either increase or decrease certain behaviors by using a structured point system and rewards. Ultimately, however, the goal is to have the individual self-control these behaviors in your absence and obtain rewards that occur naturally in the community (e.g., teacher praise, positive engagement with peers) rather than receive external rewards. For this reason, the individual should be praised and rewarded both for engaging in the target behavior *and* for accurately recording it. Once they have completed the established number of responses or intervals, they should be given access to the reward along with verbal praise, such as "I agree, you did a great job of finishing your math problems, and you remembered to mark that on your sheet." As mentioned, the baseline data will indicate where to start, which may be a small number of responses or small time periods, after which you can gradually work up to more responses or to longer time periods. This fading process increases the individual's independence, as described in the next step.

Step 6: Create Independence

To create independence, gradual and systematic fading procedures are needed. During this step, which may take place outside of your office, begin gradually and systematically fading the structured self-management program. If the individual is gathering points for discrete behaviors, such as asking a question or recording each time a question is answered, you can increase the number of responses needed before the reward is given. If they are gathering points for a behavior that is or is not occurring during a time interval, you can increase the time period while simultaneously increasing the number of points needed to receive the reward. Again, we often fade so that rewards can be provided during natural breaks in the day, such as after a class period, at recess, or even at home at the end of the day.

It is also important to ensure that the verbal prompting to engage in the behavior and to self-record is being faded. For some, it is helpful to remove the verbal prompts and provide just a visual prompt, then eventually fade the prompting altogether. At this point, some individuals can be taught to self-administer their own rewards, creating even greater independence. Self-management is a portable program designed to support behavior in the absence of a provider; therefore, any adult or provider who is helping with the program should also be faded to ensure the individual can engage in the program independently. The support person can gradually fade by leaving the classroom briefly at first and then for longer time periods and by checking in with the teacher to make sure the appropriate behavior and monitoring were accomplished during their absence. Similarly, self-management can be programmed into the natural environment without the service provider. In these settings, it will be necessary to check in with someone in that environment to make sure the desired behavior is evidenced and that accurate monitoring is taking place. Although self-management can be faded completely for most children, a small percentage will need the program to remain in place in order to be successful. If the behavior returns after the fading process, it may be necessary to reinstate the program without completely fading.

Table 6.1 provides a checklist of important variables to consider for a self-management program.

Table 6.1 Important variables for a self-management program

Is the individual eager to earn the reward? If not, reevaluate the rewards. Ultimately, we want the individual to be rewarded by natural contingencies in the environment. However, extrinsic rewards seem to be necessary initially, especially with individuals on the autism spectrum who seem less motivated by social consequences. If the individual is not enthusiastically working toward the reward, it should be reevaluated.

Does the individual clearly understand the expectations of the desired response or behavior? Often, self-management is unsuccessful because the person does not have a clear definition of what is expected. For example, one student was making a lot of distracting sounds during silent reading that disrupted the class. Instead of targeting silent reading, the interventionist chose to eliminate only one sound at a time. This confused the student, and he was not progressing. When we targeted all the sounds together and prompted him to be completely quiet, he understood the goal and immediately decreased the distracting noises.

Is the individual rarely engaging in interfering behaviors and often engaging in target behaviors while independently self-managing? With practice, the individual should be demonstrating increased success by engaging in the target behavior and self-recording independently.

Has the program been faded so that rewards occur somewhat infrequently? Over time, the goal is to fade the external rewards so that rewards more closely approximate the natural environment. For some individuals, this can be accomplished quickly; for others, more gradual steps need to be implemented for success.

Is the individual required to self-manage behavior for increasingly longer intervals (if using a wristwatch or a phone with an alarm mode) before having the opportunity to record a check mark? Steadily increasing the time intervals also helps with the fading process.

Is the individual able to self-manage behavior in your presence for extended periods of time? Once the individual is independently engaging in the desired behavior and accurately self-monitoring, you can begin fading your presence.

Is the individual able to self-manage in your absence? Self-management is designed to occur in the absence of a support person, so fading is critical. Once the individual is monitoring multiple responses or longer time intervals, the adult who implemented the self-management program should fade out. Make sure that this adult gradually and systematically leaves the individual or programs the self-management to occur in other settings in their absence.

Case Example: Jim

Jim was a young adult who talked constantly about his narrow interests of math and physics and provided excessive detail about himself.
He reported that he had few friends, which made him both depressed
and anxious in social situations. During a language sample, it was
determined that although his conversation was complex, he did not ask
any questions during conversation, even when the conversational partner gave an opening, such as "I can't wait for my vacation next month."
Although he nodded or replied with "Oh," Jim did not use questions to
continue the conversation or to show interest.

To teach Jim to ask questions during conversation, his support staff
practiced a variety of inviting statements, prompted him to respond
with a question, and then provided him with feedback after his
responses. Although he progressed quite well using this program in
a structured setting, he had difficulty generalizing it to everyday conversation. Consequently, we set up a self-management program so that
he could monitor every instance when he asked a question during conversation by using a small counter in his jacket pocket. This additional
program allowed him to serve as his own treatment provider in natural settings. After about 3 weeks of practice, asking questions began to
become second nature to him, and, in the ensuing months, his circle
of friends grew. Taking an interest in others through question-asking
was an important step to making friends and building relationships.

Other Uses of Self-Management

Combining Programs

As mentioned earlier, self-management should not be a replacement for
good teaching and using the PRT motivational components or be used
to reduce disruptive behavior without also teaching an appropriate
way to communicate. Thus, a multicomponent intervention program is
always recommended, one that includes understanding the root of the
behavior and replacing that behavior with an appropriate communicative response while ensuring that the situation is motivating for the
individual by using PRT components, whether it is at school, a work
site, or an after-school or leisure activity. However, self-management
is effective and can quickly reduce unwanted behaviors, so intervention programs often either combine self-management with other programs or use it to increase a behavior, such as a functionally equivalent
replacement behavior (FERB).

Case Example: Tam

Tam, who was fully included in a regular education kindergarten class, hit and pushed other children on the playground when he wanted attention. Although this resulted in negative attention from adults, such as being told "no hitting" and having to say "I'm sorry," these consequences were ineffective; in fact, Tam seemed to enjoy the negative attention. To avoid Tam being placed in a more restrictive setting, and for the safety of his classmates, we set up a self-management program with the goal of decreasing his aggression toward peers. At the same time, however, it was important that he also learn appropriate ways to get his peers' attention. Thus, we began the self-management with using "kind hands" for short time intervals, carefully defining the target behavior during the discrimination step and explaining that hitting and pushing were not considered to be "kind hands." We also began working on replacement behaviors. Specifically, we taught him to say "look" to gain someone's attention, to ask his peers to play (e.g., "Wanna slide?"), and to ask "Can I play?" to join an ongoing activity. These replacement behaviors took prompting over several months before Tam began using them independently, but the self-management program reduced his aggressive behaviors immediately, and he was no longer at risk for placement in a more restrictive setting. These combined programs were effective for both short- and long-term behavior improvement.

Self-Managing Replacement Behaviors

To ensure the FERB is being used in natural settings, the use of the replacement behavior can be monitored in these places. For example, one student became upset and engaged in meltdowns whenever his schoolwork became difficult. The FERB of raising his hand to get help from the teacher was targeted, and he was taught to use a counter to monitor each time he requested help instead of becoming frustrated or engaging in a meltdown. The self-management program gave him the opportunity to track the positive replacement behavior and to receive rewards, even when the teacher was assisting another student.

Feasibility

The initial steps of self-management can be time-consuming, especially when the initial intervals need to be short to create success. For most individuals who have a high level of language skills, self-management can be taught in a one-to-one setting. I often set up and show parents how to begin a self-management program during a 1-hour office appointment. Once the program is set up and the individual is showing success, parents and other providers can quickly increase the time intervals so that the program moves toward implementation in natural environments. For monitoring behavior with school-aged children, it is often helpful to have a paraprofessional, a school psychologist, or another staff member provide initial support and then gradually fade out.

Non- and Minimally Verbal Patients

Although most published self-management studies have been implemented with verbal individuals, pictorial self-management has been effectively implemented with nonverbal children. For example, one study used color pictures inserted into a photo book (Pierce and Schreibman 1994). Six to 10 of these pictures prompted everyday skills, such as setting the table, doing laundry, making the bed, and preparing food. The children were taught to self-administer rewards after completing the picture card tasks. To ensure that the children were self-managing rather than memorizing the series of steps, the order of the pictures was changed periodically. Participants learned to accurately self-monitor by flipping the card after completing the task and to self-administer their rewards independently, demonstrating the effectiveness of self-management programs for autistic children with a wide range of language abilities.

Summary

As a speech-language pathologist in the public schools, I used self-management procedures frequently with my students because I had a large caseload that allowed little time to spend with each student. Later, when working at the university, our team received several grants to explore the effectiveness of self-management procedures with autistic children. In our research and in our clinical practice, we have implemented hundreds of self-management programs across the age span from preschool to adulthood, and the rapid improvements for some students have been impressive. With the exceptionally large and increasing number of autistic patients, the supply of trained providers is limited, so procedures in which individuals are self-reliant are essential. Many teachers are not equipped to deal with behavior issues or do not have the time to prompt behaviors, and in these cases, self-management is a great tool. Self-management is both time- and cost-efficient when fading is properly implemented, and for some individuals, little overall teaching time is required. Regarding social validity ratings (i.e., when participants rate their satisfaction with and acceptability of the program), the goals, procedures, and outcomes have been evaluated as important, satisfying, and acceptable, respectively (Aljadeff-Abergel et al. 2015). The goal of any program is independence, and learning to self-manage one's own behavior is an important strategy toward that end.

References

Aljadeff-Abergel E, Schenk Y, Walmsley C, et al: The effectiveness of self-management interventions for children with autism: a literature review. Res Autism Spectr Disord 18:34–50, 2015

Carr ME: Self-management of challenging behaviours associated with autism spectrum disorder: a meta-analysis. Aust Psychol 51(4):316–333, 2016

Cihak DF, Wright R, Ayres KM: Use of self-modeling static-picture prompts via a handheld computer to facilitate self-monitoring in the general education classroom. Educ Train Autism Dev Disabil 45(1):136–149, 2010

Deitchmar C, Reeve SA, Reeve KF, et al: Incorporating video feedback into self-management training to promote generalization of social initiations by children with autism. Educ Treat Child 33(3):475–488, 2010

Ganz JB, Sigafoos J: Self-monitoring: are young adults with MR and autism able to utilize cognitive strategies independently? Educ Train Dev Disabil 40(1):24–33, 2005

Harrower JK, Dunlap G: Including children with autism in general education classrooms: a review of effective strategies. Behav Modif 25(5):762–784, 2001 11573339

Hart JE, Whalon KJ: Promote academic engagement and communication of students with autism spectrum disorder in inclusive settings. Interv Sch Clin 44(2):116–120, 2008

Koegel LK, Koegel RL, Hurley C, et al: Improving social skills and disruptive behavior in children with autism through self-management. J Appl Behav Anal 25(2):341–353, 1992 1634427

Koegel LK, Park MN, Koegel RL: Using self-management to improve the reciprocal social conversation of children with autism spectrum disorder. J Autism Dev Disord 44(5):1055–1063, 2014 24127164

Koegel RL, Koegel LK: Extended reductions in stereotypic behavior of students with autism through a self-management treatment package. J Appl Behav Anal 23(1):119–127, 1990 2335483

Newman B, Buffington DM, O'Grady MA, et al: Self-management of schedule following in three teenagers with autism. Behav Disord 20(3):190–196, 1995

Newman B, Buffington D, Hemmes N: Self-reinforcement used to increase the appropriate conversation of autistic teenagers. Education and Training in Mental Retardation and Developmental Disabilities 31:304–309, 1996

Palmen A, Didden R, Arts M: Improving question asking in high-functioning adolescents with autism spectrum disorders: effectiveness of small-group training. Autism 12(1):83–98, 2008 18178598

Pierce KL, Schreibman L: Teaching daily living skills to children with autism in unsupervised settings through pictorial self-management. J Appl Behav Anal 27(3):471–481, 1994 7928790

Reinecke DR, Newman B, Meinberg DL: Self-management of sharing in three pre-schoolers with autism. Education and Training in Mental Retardation and Developmental Disabilities 34(3):312–317, 1999

Simmons CA, Ardoin SP, Ayres KM, et al: Parent-implemented self-management intervention on the on-task behavior of students with autism. Sch Psychol 37(3):273–284, 2022 35324235

Stahmer AC, Schreibman L: Teaching children with autism appropriate play in unsupervised environments using a self-management treatment package. J Appl Behav Anal 25(2):447–459,1992 1634432

7

Social Engagement Across the Lifespan

Friends and Relationships

Contrary to popular misconceptions, individuals with autism report that they want friends, romantic relationships, and close connections with loved ones (Bennett et al. 2018), an important fact for psychiatrists and providers to be aware of and to discuss with parents and providers. Socialization is critical for improved outcomes in adulthood; however, this area is too often neglected, especially in schools that allow autistic children to wander the playground alone despite a plethora of available peers to draw from for social activities. Although important and desired, socialization can be challenging for many on the autism spectrum because of their communicative difficulties, and most will need support in this area to ensure success. Chatting, initiating contact, and solving disagreements are all social communicative areas that are reported to be more challenging for this population (Finke 2023). In this chapter, I describe specific ways pivotal response treatment (PRT) has been implemented in infancy, elementary school, middle and high school, college, and beyond to support and teach socialization using motivational contexts.

Although friendships evolve throughout the lifespan, socialization begins very early on. In the first years of life, neurotypical children will engage in reciprocal interactions with peers that consider the other child's perspective. During these early interactions, conflicts are usually moderated by parent and peer reactions, and the support provided by parents can influence future interactions. During the elementary school years and preadolescence, friendships assist with developing an awareness of social rules, a sense of belonging and value from non-family individuals, and acceptance. In adolescence, more time is spent with peers, creating independence from parents and increased intimacy (O'Connor et al. 2022). Over time, friendships can provide social support in terms of feeling part of a community and having someone to connect with for help, information, and feedback. Friendships can play a large role in an individual's mental health and overall well-being and can provide a buffer against inequalities, including bullying, loneliness, and social rejection. Unfortunately, some friendships support unwanted and dangerous behaviors, so monitoring and guidance are imperative, especially with individuals who are naïve or trusting or lack experience in the social world.

Research has studied areas such as number of friends, best friends, and the quality of friendships; however, how friendship is defined and the value individuals place on friendships vary widely (Lu et al. 2021). Unfortunately, individuals with autism spectrum disorder have been shown to have fewer and lower-quality friendships than their neurotypical peers, as reported by parents, self-report, and sociometric measures (Mendelson et al. 2016). They also are rarely listed on classmates' top friendship lists. Thus, compared with neurotypical children, who develop friendships without support, children on the autism spectrum generally require explicit education in socialization.

Support for Socialization

When providing intervention and support for social areas, many programs work on social goals in an isolated setting with adults, such as the speech-language pathologist, psychologist, or applied behavior analysis provider. Adult-child interactions are very different from child-child interactions. Adults tend to initiate interactions with autistic children and create highly responsive and anticipatory social environments. On the other hand, child-child interactions are more balanced, with nearly equal involvement expected. For this reason, many children on the autism spectrum spend more time with adults than their peers and may show greater social competence with adults than peers. Unfortunately, early social isolation from peers may escalate and increase social challenges as a child grows, later affecting peer acceptance and quality of life (L.K. Koegel et al. 2001). Furthermore, although neurotypical and autistic children engage in a similar number of interactions with adults, peer-peer interactions for autistic children are very low or frequently nonexistent, regardless of their communicative or cognitive level (L.K. Koegel et al. 2001). Children with autism initiate interactions less frequently than their peers and are often unresponsive to peers' initiations (Fedewa et al. 2024). Thus, social interventions with peers are critical from an early age. Fortunately, several programs have resulted in improvements in peer-peer interactions, beginning at the preschool age level and continuing throughout the lifespan. These can be particularly helpful if the PRT motivational components are incorporated. Some important considerations for such programs include

- **Natural settings.** Social intervention should take place in natural settings. Pulling a child out of class or recess or providing intervention in an isolated setting often only results in challenges with generalization.
- **Neurotypical peers.** Children on the autism spectrum perform better when they are with neurotypical peers who can serve as role models and assist with prompting and supporting newly learned social behaviors. If a child does not have access to neurotypical peers, such as children placed in a special education classroom, participation in recreational and afterschool or weekend programs or recruitment of neurotypical peers from other settings can be helpful for providing environments for peer interactions.
- **Child choice.** Incorporating the autistic child's interests into the social activity helps greatly with improving their engagement and socialization across the lifespan. Some interests may need to be adjusted a bit to be more age-appropriate and relevant to their neurotypical peers.
- **Peer mediation.** Many effective interventions actively recruit peers and provide them with explicit procedures to teach and support socialization of the autistic child. These have been shown to be effective from preschool through adulthood.
- **Multicomponent interventions.** A single intervention program usually is not sufficient for making substantial gains in

socialization. A multicomponent program that focuses on the child with autism, peer supports, and creating an environment that is conducive to socialization (e.g., seating arrangements with preferred peers, clubs and activities) is often needed.

- **Practice, practice, practice.** Although many school programs state that children with autism need a "break" during recess and other unstructured engagement periods, intervention during this valuable time with peers is critical. Like any activity, the more supported and guided practice a child receives, the more competent with socialization they will become.

Improving Play Using PRT

PRT strategies have been used to improve play in 5- to 9-year-olds by choosing preferred toys, modeling sociodramatic play, and then providing the desired toy when the child engages in the dramatic play. For example, if a child chooses to play with a doctor's kit, the interventionist may model making a phone call to the doctor. Once the child pretends to call the doctor, they are given the doctor kit as a natural reward. Similarly, if the child chooses to play with toy foods, the support provider might model an eating or cooking activity. If the child imitates the model or makes another attempt or response related to the food theme, they would be naturally rewarded with the food items. Research shows that following two or three sessions per week for a total of 16 hours of support, children improved their role-playing, make-believe play, persistence in carrying through a play theme, and spontaneous communication. Time engaged in social and verbal behaviors also increased. Some children's social gains and all communication gains generalized to new settings and new play partners. Follow-up probes showed continued improvement in all areas compared with pretreatment measures (Thorp et al. 1995).

A randomized controlled study used PRT to teach 4- to 6-year-olds to make social, initiated requests to neurotypical peers, who were prompted to reward these attempts during free play and snack time (Gengoux et al. 2021). Following 8 weeks of weekly 75-minute group sessions, the PRT group showed significantly greater social initiations compared with the group receiving treatment as usual (TAU). Additionally, following this intervention, the PRT group's joint attention and social interaction with peers also improved, even though these areas were not specifically targeted during the intervention.

Furthermore, the PRT group showed greater improvements on global measures of social communication, whereas the TAU group was scored as largely unchanged by naïve observers. Although this study focused on only one communicative function, requests (e.g., "Pass the juice, please," "Can I have a glue stick?"), the generalization to joint attention and engagement provides optimism that focusing on the PRT components of child choice and teaching peers to provide natural rewards will lead to widespread improvement in socialization for young children.

Another study recruited third-grade peers to use PRT procedures to improve play with autistic children who rarely or never interacted with peers. The peers were given written and pictorial instructions. Their training included getting the child's attention, offering choices, varying the activities according to the autistic peer's preferences, modeling appropriate social and verbal behaviors (e.g., making positive statements and acting out scripts), rewarding attempts, encouraging and extending verbalizations (e.g., providing toys contingent upon verbalizations), asking questions, taking turns, narrating, and providing more complex language models. The procedures were modeled by an adult during four 30-minute sessions over a 2-week period, followed by some direct feedback with the autistic child and peer. Following the training, the autistic children showed improvements in their social and verbal interactions, including word use and sentence length. Untargeted joint attention and initiated play interactions also improved. These gains continued at a 2-month postintervention follow-up (Pierce and Schreibman 1995).

Another study replicated findings that PRT implemented by peers can improve socialization in 7- and 8-year-old boys on the autism spectrum who had intellectual and communicative disabilities and rarely or never interacted with peers (Pierce and Schreibman 1997). With the help of their trained peers, the autistic boys improved their quality and quantity of peer social communication. An important finding of this study was that if multiple peers are taught to implement PRT, children on the autism spectrum seem likely to generalize their socialization gains to new and untrained peers. This suggests the widespread benefits of teaching PRT to groups of peers who interact with children on the autism spectrum. It also suggests more positive outcomes when the autistic child has opportunities to practice with multiple skilled peers rather than just one trained peer. Overall, providing PRT training to peers appears to be a particularly helpful and cost-efficient method for improving social communication and engagement.

PRT for Improving Socialization in Adolescence

PRT procedures can also improve socialization during adolescence. Opportunities for peer social interaction can be implemented during lunch periods, using the adolescent's preferred interests (R. Koegel et al. 2013). An existing club around the autistic student's interests can be used or developed; a specialist or teacher who knows the child well can create the club and invite other interested peers. Such clubs can be advertised to the school through intercom announcements, flyers, and teacher announcements, just like other clubs. Interest-focused clubs have been shown to be effective with older elementary, middle, and high school students, reversing the pattern of these students spending most or all of their time socially isolated (L.K. Koegel et al. 2001, 2012; R. Koegel et al. 2012, 2013).

A particular advantage of arranging activities or clubs around the student's preferred interests is that many autistic individuals have already acquired a large amount of information on the topic, and thus they are often considered the most valued peer in the club. The following are some examples of school clubs that have been successfully implemented using the PRT motivational components.

Case Example: Manual

> High school student Manual spent lunchtime alone and isolated from peers. At home, he enjoyed movies and remembered details about each, including the actors, lines, and credits. His school did not have any type of movie club, so a movie trivia club was created for him. Two teams were formed, and short clips of popular movies were played. The students were asked to answer questions about the movies, and the team with the most points was awarded movie tickets. Unsurprisingly, Manual's team always won the competitions because his knowledge on the topic was so profound. Consequently, his peers always asked him to be on their team, and his newly formed group of friends enjoyed going to the movies with their prize tickets and hanging out afterward.

Case Example: Jordan

> Jordan attended middle school. Although she often sat at a table with peers, she never interacted with them. She enjoyed cooking, so a cooking club during lunchtime was created that used no-bake recipes the

students could prepare and immediately enjoy. Students were grouped by task and engaged in considerable social communication to cooperatively prepare the food. Without specific intervention, this club resulted in 100% engagement between Jordan and her peers during lunch, and her social verbal initiations and responses greatly increased. She often spent her cooking periods laughing and smiling, in contrast to previously, when she was unengaged and sullen.

Case Example: Clay

Clay was a middle school student who was relentlessly teased by his peers. He ate alone and did not interact with his peers, but they often made inappropriate and rude comments to him while passing by. At home, he spent most of his free time drawing and had become quite a skilled artist. He could draw vehicles and buildings to scale and perspective, a challenge for his classmates. His art teacher created a drawing club at lunch and appointed him as her assistant. She taught him how to explain principles of drawing to his peers and provide them with encouraging feedback. He was fully engaged during each club, beginning from the very first meeting, and was valued as a mentor to other members, who constantly asked him questions and sought his help. This provided him with confidence, individuals with whom he could interact regularly, and frequent praise and compliments from his peers.

When these clubs around the student's interests are established, we see increases in engagement and verbal initiations, as well as increased opportunities for friendships to develop (L.K. Koegel et al. 2012; R. Koegel et al. 2013). Some schools may have many existing clubs for students to choose from, whereas other schools may need to create a club that interests the autistic student and peers. Development of and participation in clubs can be written into the student's individualized education program for implementation by a speech-language pathologist, school psychologist, or special or regular education teacher. Clubs also have been run successfully by parents and college students. Although most children demonstrate social improvements simply by attending the clubs around their interests, peers in the club can be recruited to help with specific goals for the autistic child, such as prompting the student to ask questions, repeating a question if the student did not respond, or supporting them in providing directions or information, particularly if the autistic student has communication challenges.

The importance of social engagement cannot be understated. Building good peer relations can create long-lasting gains that cannot be achieved in adult-child relationships, and despite finding them challenging, autistic adolescents report the desire and yearning for peer relationships. Peers, with supervision and feedback, can be effective supports in assisting with implementing goals.

PRT for Improving Socialization in Adulthood

After graduating from high school, many autistic adults find themselves isolated from peers. PRT procedures for encouraging engagement also have been effective with college students and young adults. For example, similarly aged peer mentor volunteers working collaboratively with a skilled clinician can accompany autistic college students or young adults to school clubs or community activities that appeal to their interests (Ashbaugh et al. 2017). College settings are ideal for social opportunities because most students have left their cliques of friends and are searching for new ones. Many colleges also offer a large number and wide range of extracurricular clubs for students to join. Encouraging autistic college students to attend clubs around their interests can be an excellent way to help them meet other like-minded students. Optional peer support may be requested by the autistic adult and can be arranged by recruiting a neurotypical peer to attend the clubs as well. Autistic college students who engage in these supported activities report higher life satisfaction and quality and engage in a larger number of social events outside of the club meetings (L.K. Koegel et al. 2013).

Case Example: Dylan

> Dylan's college had a club devoted to anime, one of his favorite forms of entertainment. Dylan expressed anxiety at attending a club on his own, so a peer mentor (a psychology student interested in studying autism) was selected to accompany him. During the club meetings, Dylan interacted with another attendee and enjoyed her company so much that they began going on outings together outside of the club, which provided him with opportunities to meet additional peers. Dylan's father attempted to be helpful and made business cards for him; however, when Dylan began to hand out business cards at the next club meeting, his peer mentor provided feedback that young people put numbers into their phones and do not hand out business cards.

His peer mentor was able to support Dylan in real situations that would
be difficult, if not impossible, to teach outside of a natural setting.

Case Example: Ezekiel

Ezekiel finished high school and had a part-time job but did not engage
with peers. He lived at home, and both of his parents worked full-time,
so he spent most of the day alone playing computer games. During
an initial meeting, he expressed an interest in dancing. His town had
a community dance class, so he signed up for a beginning class and
attended with a peer mentor. Fortuitously, the teacher often had the
students change partners, so Ezekiel was able to meet new people naturally within the dance activities. His mentor practiced having him
ask questions and compliment other club members, and soon he had a
group of friends to dance and hang out with outside of class.

Case Example: Lety

Lety was a college student who reported being depressed because she
did not have friends. Although she had a roommate, they rarely interacted. Lety was interested in animals, and because there were very
few animals on campus, an animal shelter close to her school was con-
tacted. The shelter needed volunteers, so Lety and her peer mentor took
advantage of the opportunity to walk and socialize the animals. After
seeing her caring nature, the shelter asked her to assist with locating
adoptive families and to volunteer at their spay and neuter clinic. This
provided Lety with a variety of opportunities to develop friendships
with other animal lovers.

Individual support programs for individuals with social challenges
are often implemented to accompany these social clubs and outings
(Ashbaugh et al. 2017). Peer mentors can discreetly prompt targeted
areas in these natural settings. For example, if the autistic adult does
not ask many questions, the peer mentor can subtly prompt a question
in the moment by saying, "I wonder what classes everyone is taking."
They can also prompt questions before the event, such as "Don't for-
get to ask everyone what classes they're taking and what their favorite
classes are." Research also shows that when college students engage
socially in school clubs, their grades are positively affected and other
nonstructured social activities with peers increase outside of the desig-
nated club times, again attesting to the widespread positive outcomes
of supported social activities (Ashbaugh et al. 2017).

PRT, Robots, and Artificial Intelligence

PRT to improve social communication has also been studied using various types of artificial intelligence (AI). For example, robots have been programmed to provide individualized instruction in asking questions, using longer utterances, responding to more complex utterances, protesting, and requesting. When affect is measured, the children seem to enjoy the sessions and exhibit high motivation. These games and other enjoyable activities using a robot have the potential to result in gains over time as they continue to be refined (van den Berk-Smeekens et al. 2022). In addition, most parents report that this type of intervention is a very acceptable method of support for their children (van den Berk-Smeekens et al. 2020).

Preliminary research also suggests that AI applications can be effective at improving social conversation in various areas (Koegel et. al. 2025), including increasing verbal empathetic responses, asking more questions, talking the right amount, understanding sarcasm, giving compliments, making relevant responses, and so on, that previously required face-to-face interventions.[1] These AI options allow individuals to practice social skills in the privacy of their own homes and can offer support when a provider is not available. AI has the potential to support busy parents by providing additional opportunities for independent practice in the absence of a parent or treatment provider. However, many available AI programs have not yet been empirically validated; thus, careful attention to the evidence base is warranted for programs claiming to improve outcomes in this population.

Summary

Across the age span, developing social relationships and friendships has been discussed as an important and necessary part of development that leads to positive self-value and self-esteem, as well as psychosocial well-being. In contrast, fewer and lower-quality friendships can lead to depression and anxiety (O'Connor et al. 2022). Because challenges with social engagement often result in later-diagnosed social anxiety (Stark

---

[1] Stanford University Collaborative AI autism research project between the School of Medicine and the Computer Science Department. Contact: Lynnk@Stanford.edu. See also L.K. Koegel et al. 2025.

et al. 2023), and a low or perceived unsatisfactory number of social activities can lead to loneliness and depression (Adams et al. 2024), there is an urgent need to

1) Create and implement programs that offer opportunities for socialization by focusing on the preferred interests of autistic individuals across the age span. Programs can be implemented throughout the day in various settings to improve and enhance socialization.
2) Support these social activities with supplemental services, including peer-mediated support, peer mentors, and targeted interventions.
3) Work with the broader neurotypical community to understand and embrace human differences, reduce bullying, and encourage inclusion. Autistic individuals experience widespread discrimination, bullying, and exclusion that can lead to further mental health conditions and unemployment.
4) Provide cognitive-behavioral therapy and other evidence-based interventions simultaneously to reduce any co-occurring conditions.

Improved education and support for autistic individuals and the greater community are long overdue. Psychiatrists and other providers must address socialization at the earliest possible point in time and suggest a variety of supports that will improve autistic individuals' social contacts, peer interactions, recreational activities, and community engagement. Opportunities for socialization should be written into individualized education programs and adult service plans, and autism training programs aimed at improving socialization should be a part of every school and community program. Without such support, autistic individuals will have a lifelong disadvantage.

References

Adams RE, Lampinen L, Zheng S, et al: Associations between social activities and depressive symptoms in adolescents and young adults with autism spectrum disorder: testing the indirect effects of loneliness. Autism 28(2):461–473, 2024 37212127

Ashbaugh K, Koegel R, Koegel L: Increasing social integration for college students with autism spectrum disorder. Behav Dev Bull 22(1):183–196, 2017 28642808

Bennett M, Webster AA, Goodall E, et al: Establishing social inclusion the autism way: denying the "they don't want friends" myth, in Life on the Autism Spectrum: Translating Myths and Misconceptions Into Positive Futures. New York, Springer, 2018, pp 173–193

Fedewa M, Watkins L, Barnard-Brak L, et al: A systematic review and meta-analysis of single case experimental design play interventions for children with autism and their peers. Rev J Autism Dev Disord 11(2):361–383, 2024

Finke EH: The kind of friend I think I am: perceptions of autistic and non-autistic young adults. J Autism Dev Disord 53(8):3047–3064, 2023 35570241

Gengoux GW, Schwartzman JM, Millan ME, et al: Enhancing social initiations using naturalistic behavioral intervention: outcomes from a randomized controlled trial for children with autism. J Autism Dev Disord 51(10):3547–3563, 2021 33387236

Koegel LK, Koegel RL, Frea WD, et al: Identifying early intervention targets for children with autism in inclusive school settings. Behav Modif 25(5):745–761, 2001 11573338

Koegel LK, Vernon T, Koegel RL, et al: Improving social engagement and initiations between children with autism spectrum disorder and their peers in inclusive settings. J Posit Behav Interv 14(4):220–227, 2012 25328380

Koegel LK, Ashbaugh K, Koegel RL, et al: Increasing socialization in adults with Asperger's syndrome. Psychol Sch 50(9):899–909, 2013

Koegel LK, Ponder E, Bruzzese T, et al: Using artificial intelligence to improve empathetic statements in autistic adolescents and adults: a randomized clinical trial. J Autism Dev Disord 2025 [Epub ahead of print]

Koegel R, Fredeen R, Kim S, et al: Using perseverative interests to improve interactions between adolescents with autism and their typical peers in school settings. J Posit Behav Interv 14(3):133–141, 2012 24163577

Koegel R, Kim S, Koegel L, et al: Improving socialization for high school students with ASD by using their preferred interests. J Autism Dev Disord 43(9):2121–2134, 2013 23361918

Lu P, Oh J, Leahy KE, et al: Friendship importance around the world: links to cultural factors, health, and well-being. Front Psychol 11:570839, 2021 33536962

Mendelson JL, Gates JA, Lerner MD: Friendship in school-age boys with autism spectrum disorders: a meta-analytic summary and developmental, process-based model. Psychol Bull 142(6):601–622, 2016 26752425

O'Connor RAG, van den Bedem N, Blijd-Hoogewys EMA, et al: Friendship quality among autistic and non-autistic (pre-) adolescents: protective or risk factor for mental health? Autism 26(8):2041–2051, 2022 35068188

Pierce K, Schreibman L: Increasing complex social behaviors in children with autism: effects of peer-implemented pivotal response training. J Appl Behav Anal 28(3):285–295, 1995 7592145

Pierce K, Schreibman L: Multiple peer use of pivotal response training to increase social behaviors of classmates with autism: results from trained and untrained peers. J Appl Behav Anal 30(1):157–160, 1997 9103991

Stark C, Groves NB, Kofler MJ: Is reduced social competence a mechanism linking elevated autism spectrum symptoms with increased risk for social anxiety? Br J Clin Psychol 62(1):129–145, 2023 36300947

Thorp DM, Stahmer AC, Schreibman L: Effects of sociodramatic play training on children with autism. J Autism Dev Disord 25(3):265–282, 1995 7559292

van den Berk-Smeekens I, van Dongen-Boomsma M, De Korte MWP, et al: Adherence and acceptability of a robot-assisted pivotal response treatment protocol for children with autism spectrum disorder. Sci Rep 10(1):8110, 2020 32415231

van den Berk-Smeekens I, de Korte MWP, van Dongen-Boomsma M, et al: Pivotal response treatment with and without robot-assistance for children with autism: a randomized controlled trial. Eur Child Adolesc Psychiatry 31(12):1871–1883, 2022 34106357

Improving Social Conversation

In this chapter, I discuss how to assess and provide recommendations for improving specific social conversational areas that are challenging for autistic individuals. Some individuals on the autism spectrum are perfectly content with their social conversation skills, but others many find that challenges in this area lead to difficulties with dating, employment, interpersonal relationships, and intimate relationships. Across the lifespan, most autistic individuals have smaller social networks, fewer close friends, and lower participation in community activities despite their longing for casual and intimate relationships (Chang and Dean 2022). Furthermore, some autistic adults who are verbal report "masking" or "camouflaging" by hiding behaviors that may be considered socially unacceptable and attempting to engage in "acceptable" social behaviors. Although masking may be helpful for some, it can be draining, stressful, and exhausting for others. Research in this area and into the extent to which it leads to co-occurring mental health conditions, and even suicide, is lacking and needed (Cremone et al. 2023).

Unfortunately, many autistic individuals develop social anxiety and depression as a direct consequence of the social communication challenges inherent to an autism diagnosis. Fewer social relationships may lead to loneliness, which in turn can cause emotional distress, anxiety, and depression (Hymas et al. 2022). Although nonautistic individuals may also experience loneliness, the continual effect of loneliness over time can produce significant mental health issues. Autistic individuals also are more likely to be bullied and victimized; research shows that social and communication challenges, such as not being attuned to the daily social situation, can result in increased levels of bullying (Forrest et al. 2020). Bullying needs to be addressed from both sides, not only by reducing intolerable aggressive acts by bullies but also by simultaneously targeting social communication in individuals on the autism spectrum.

Social conversation can be assessed during office visits by conversing with the patient and probing for certain responses and behaviors. The conversational partner can provide opportunities that evoke particular responses for specific areas that can be challenging for individuals on the autism spectrum.

Challenges and Assessment

Empathy

For many years, individuals with autism have been described as lacking empathy or having deficits in theory of mind because they have difficulties relating to and reflecting on the mental states of others. A diagnostic characteristic of autism spectrum disorder (ASD), as stated in DSM-5 (American Psychiatric Association 2022), is a reduced sharing of interests, emotions, or affect, along with a failure to initiate or respond to social interactions. Some individuals have attempted to depathologize autism and have discussed the *double empathy theory*, which suggests that the breakdown in empathy can be bidirectional between individuals with and those without autism—that is, problems arise when the autistic individual does not understand social norms and the neurotypical conversational partner does not understand the unique difficulties of ASD. However, for autistic individuals who desire to improve their skills in this area, some interventions have been successful.

Assessment

To assess this area, we provide opportunities for the individual to respond with verbal empathy in social conversation. For example, we provide leading statements that usually prompt an empathetic response. We do this with both positive and negative statements and then pause for a few seconds after each to wait for a response. For example, the assessor might say, "I'm so excited about the weekend. My sister is visiting, and I haven't seen her in so long." If the autistic individual responds with "I'm doing something fun this weekend, too," this does not show an interest in the other person's happiness. Similarly, if the assessor says, "I strained my calf exercising, and it's really been hurting," and the response is "Uh-huh" or "Oh," this again indicates that the individual may need support with improving empathetic responses. These types of leading statements can be sprinkled throughout the natural conversation to get an idea of the individual's use of verbal empathetic responses.

Treatment

Once you have a good idea of whether the individual has challenges expressing verbal empathetic statements, and after ensuring that they desire to improve their social conversation, you can begin targeting this area. It is usually helpful to start by providing a schematic for the individual. This may appear with the general categories and examples as shown in Table 8.1.

Various statements of emotion can be expressed, and the schematic can be used as a visual prompt (by pointing to each response of expressing understanding and asking a question). With practice, coming up with these types of responses becomes easier, and individuals respond more readily. The session can be video recorded and discussed afterward (L.K. Koegel et al. 2016a), or the individual can be provided with a checklist to mark off each category as a self-management system if additional support is desired. As the individual begins using these empathetic responses during conversation, the schematic and boxes can be faded.

Case Example: Arthur

> Arthur was a high-achieving college student but reported that he was having difficulty at his part-time job on campus. He stated that coworkers did not include him in conversations and appeared to avoid him during breaks. An observation of his social conversation showed that his responses to another person's emotion were related to his own situations. For example, when someone said, "I got a really bad grade on my English test," he responded with "I got an 'A' on my English test, but I studied really hard." When a coworker said, "I went on a great

Table 8.1 Schematic (prompting) for improving verbal empathetic responses

Statement of emotion	Express understanding	Show interest with a question
[Stress] I have a test tomorrow.	Tests can be so stressful.	Do you feel like you'll do okay on it?
[Sick] I have a sore throat today.	I'm sorry to hear that.	Have you seen a doctor?
[Excited] I can't wait for the weekend because my sister is visiting.	That sounds like fun.	What are you going to do?

hike on Saturday," he responded with "Finals are coming up so everyone should be home studying, not going to parties." After several treatment sessions using the schematic, Arthur quickly learned empathetic responses to these statements, such as "English tests can be really hard. Would you like to study with me?" or "Hiking is great. Where did you go?" This simple adjustment in his verbal empathetic responses made a notable difference in his conversation and led to success in improving his social engagement with other students. In fact, shortly after the treatment was implemented, he reported dating a college classmate.

Question-Asking

Chapter 3, "The Importance of Initiations," described ways to increase or instate question-asking. Many individuals on the autism spectrum are quite competent with asking questions but may have challenges using questions during conversation.

Responding With a Question

Assessment

Assessing question-asking can be accomplished during a simple conversation in your office, via telehealth, or by observing the patient with another person. Many autistic individuals ask too few or no questions during social conversation. To assess this, you can provide leading statements that beg a question. For example, during the conversation, you might say, "I had a great weekend," "My friend is visiting this weekend," or "I'm going to a new restaurant tonight"—statements about which another person would likely ask questions. Be sure to provide pauses after the statements to give the individual a chance to respond.

Treatment

If the individual does not ask a question in response to the leading statement, this can be prompted; for example, after saying, "I had a great weekend," you can prompt a follow-up question by saying, "A good question to ask me would be 'What did you do?'" The prompt can be verbal or written. For example, you could hold up a piece of paper that says "Ask a question," or if the patient needs a more supportive prompt, it could say "Where," "Who," or "What" (Doggett et al. 2013) or even include the full question to start. Frequent practice with asking questions can be helpful, remembering that prompting should be gradually faded so that the questions are eventually asked spontaneously and naturally during conversation.

Case Example: Gene

> Gene was an intelligent and good-looking young man who attended an Ivy League university. He had a small group of friends in his private high school but was having trouble making friends in college. Although he had asked out and taken several women on first dates during the early months of school, none of the women had ever agreed to a second date. This caused Gene considerable depression, and he resorted to staying up most of the night playing video games and missing many of his classes. He sought professional help from a psychologist, who simply asked him, "Why don't you think you have friends?" which he was unable to answer. He also confided that he had considered suicide because of his loneliness and lack of friends. During a conversation sample, it was noted that he asked zero questions. Although he nodded during pauses and at appropriate times for a question, he did not respond verbally. After four sessions practicing with questions, Gene was able to verbally express his interest in others and soon thereafter began steadily dating a fellow student. This practical intervention made a huge difference for him.

Initiating a Question

Treatment

Initiating questions is another challenging area for many individuals. A helpful intervention for improving this skill is the use of question banks (Koegel et al. 2021). This involves working with the individual to develop a list of questions (we usually shoot for 50) and having them practice asking those questions. During the practice sessions, the provider works with the individual to ensure that the questions are appropriate and comfortable for them to initiate (e.g., "Where were you born?"; "Do you have any sisters or brothers?"; "Are you reading any good books?"; "Have you watched any good movies lately?"; "What did you do over the weekend?"). If any questions relate to gender or politics or are too personal (e.g., "Are you male or female?"; "What is your sexual preference?"; "Who did you vote for in the last election?"), the individual is provided with feedback, and the question is not included in the bank.

Next, each question is printed on an individual card. The individual reads the card silently, then looks at the support provider and asks the question. They should then continue to look at the conversational partner while listening to the answer. Our research shows that after only four half-hour sessions, individuals were able to improve their social interactions during conversations by initiating questions to others (Koegel et al. 2021). This simple strategy can be combined with others to improve initiated conversation with peers. It has been effective with individuals who interact infrequently, giving them a strategy for starting a conversation, and provides variation for those who ask the same questions repetitively as a way of engaging with others.

Case Example: Genevieve

> Genevieve was a high school student who enjoyed interacting with others but repeatedly asked her peers the same questions, such as "What's your favorite color?" or "What's your favorite food?" Although it was encouraging that she wanted to socially interact, we thought her conversation would be improved if she initiated different questions. Therefore, we used the question bank treatment, and after just 4 weeks of practice, she began to initiate a large variety of different questions with peers, leading to much more responsiveness and richer conversations.

Increasing Positive Statements

For the subgroup of individuals who make repeated negative statements during social interactions, positive reframing can be taught. To do this, a combination of self-management and video feedback can be used (Koegel et al. 2016b).

Assessment

The percentage of positive and negative statements someone uses can be measured during a short conversation sample. If their conversation is too negative, support in this area can be helpful.

Treatment

First, we provide psychoeducation by describing the advantages of reframing and how excessive negative statements can affect friendships and relationships with coworkers, family members, peers, and employers. Next, we select negative statements that the autistic individual used during our conversation, and we discuss how the statements could be reframed to be more positive. For example, we might say, "Instead of saying you hate school and can't wait to be done with the school year, a positive way of saying the same thing might be 'I'm really looking forward to summer.'" Following this, we check in to confirm that the individual would like to improve this area.

For treatment, video feedback is used. Specifically, a conversation between the patient and the treatment provider or a peer is video recorded. Next, the provider watches the conversation with the patient and pauses after each statement or question by the conversational partner that receives a negative response from the patient. The autistic individual is then asked to provide three responses that are positively reframed and to explain why each response is positive or neutral (not negative). At least 6 statements or questions are played, giving the individual an opportunity to create a total of 18 positive or neutral responses. Following these sessions, conversation probes are collected. During these probes, the individual is asked to self-manage their positive statements by making a check mark on a sheet of paper or pressing a counter following each minute in which only positive or neutral responses are made (i.e., minutes without negative statements). When the autistic individual can independently produce three positive/neutral statements for each opportunity during the practice portion of the sessions, and conversational probes show that negative responses are reduced to 10% or lower over five consecutive probes, the video modeling is faded. At this point, probes with independent peers in community settings are collected. If the individual continues to use the positively reframed responses (i.e., no negative statements), the intervention is considered complete.

Research shows that this intervention is effective in greatly decreasing or eliminating negative statements with generalization and maintenance. Following treatment, almost all autistic adolescents and adults show improvements in positive affect and interest and are scored as being more socially desirable to peers during conversation. On standardized measures of depression, most of the autistic individuals report lower depression, anxiety, and helplessness following the intervention, and almost all these gains are maintained at follow-up (Koegel et al. 2016b).

Case Example: Maverick

> Maverick worked at an office while in college. When coworkers greeted him or engaged him in small talk, he would begin a diatribe about how stressed he was about school, the new rash he had, how he had not slept well, and many other negative responses. In fact, a casual "How's it going?" usually resulted in the response of "Horrible!" Over time, coworkers avoided him or passed by him without interacting. It was suggested that Maverick begin treatment for positive reframing, to which he agreed. In fact, he was unaware of how many negative comments he made until he began watching the video clips. The treatment was effective, and within a few months, Maverick began responding positively. He reported reduced social isolation, improved happiness, and less social anxiety following the treatment.

Talking the Right Amount

Some autistic individuals talk too much or too little. Responding with one-word answers does not lead to an engaged reciprocal conversation, and responding with too many details can interfere with the listener's attention. Feedback and instruction on providing the right amount of information can be helpful in improving social conversation.

Assessment

Assessing the length of responses and the amount of information provided can be accomplished during a short conversation. It is helpful to ask general questions in addition to questions about the patient's strong interests. Often, responses vary with the conversation topic. If the person answers with one-word responses or provides lengthy, detailed responses with too much information, treatment in this area should be helpful.

Treatment

Using a schematic can be helpful for prompting the autistic individual to respond with the right amount of detail. A suggested schematic uses three circles with arrows in between (Figure 8.1). In the first circle, we write "Answer the question," in the second, "Add information," and in the third, "Ask a question." For individuals who provide too little information, we add an extra circle before "Ask a question" that says "Add more information." We practice this first by demonstrating; for example, I might say, "If someone asks how my weekend was, I can respond with 'It was great' [while pointing to the first circle]; 'I went hiking with my sister in the Baylands Nature Preserve' [while pointing to the second circle]; 'How about you, what did you do this weekend?' [while pointing to the third circle]."

Next, we practice with the schematic by asking questions, pointing to the circles, and having the autistic individual tally their own number of correct responses. This essentially combines the schematic with self-management. After 9–16 practice sessions, adolescents and adults can improve their reciprocal conversation by talking the right amount and are scored by independent observers as appearing more socially competent and interesting, having improved reciprocity, and being more natural in their social interactions (L.K. Koegel et al. 2014).

Case Example: Austin

Austin, an adolescent, was very interested in rocks and gems and had acquired a large amount of information about them. He tended to give long lectures on the topic, including what minerals composed a

Figure 8.1 Schematic for visually prompting the right amount of talking.

specific gemstone, the history of the stone (e.g., when it was first found, what it symbolized), the rarity of the gem, the birthstone month, the price, the range of sizes, and any other facts he knew. Although any one or two of these facts could be interesting, hearing dozens of them made the conversational partner lose interest. After just a few sessions, Austin learned to monitor himself and provide just one or two facts about a stone (or any other topic) before asking a question. By limiting the details he provided, he kept the conversational partner's interest and attention, and his question-asking kept the conversation balanced by allowing equal talking space for the conversational partner. After a few months of weekly sessions and follow-through by his parents, Austin learned to have balanced back-and-forth conversations. Follow-up assessment 1 year posttreatment showed that he had maintained his gains.

Case Example: Sam

Sam, a young adult, indicated that he wanted friends, but when asked a question, he responded with one-word answers or short phrases. For example, if someone said, "Hey, how are you?" he responded with "Fine." His responses to open-ended questions, such as "What did you do over the weekend?" were generally very short, such as "Not much." He never provided additional information and did not respond with reciprocal questions. Using the schematic and self-management, we practiced asking him questions (e.g., "How are you?") and having him respond, add an additional piece of information, and ask a question. For example, "I'm great. I love this sunny weather. How are you doing?" or, in response to a question about his weekend: "I just relaxed and did some homework. I had a lot of math, but it was easy. How was your weekend?" A few months' practice with providing longer responses and asking a follow-up question made a huge difference in his social conversation.

Greetings and Departures

Other areas that can lead to improved conversation through practice are greetings and departures. We generally try to have the autistic individual make eye contact (if someone expresses discomfort with making eye contact, looking at the forehead is usually more comfortable and appears as good eye contact to the communicative partner) and, once they have spoken a simple word of greeting, ask a question that will continue the conversation. For example, if someone says, "Hi," instead of replying only with another "Hi," a question can be added to keep the conversation going: "Hi, how have you been?" or "Hi, what have you been up to?" For departures, we prompt the autistic individual to make a polite statement. Instead of saying only "Okay" or "Bye" when someone is departing, adding "It was nice seeing you" or "It was nice chatting with you" makes the exit friendlier. These often need to be practiced until they are used regularly.

Case Example: Bill

> Bill started a new job but reported difficulty meeting coworkers. It was noted that he responded by saying only "Hi!" when others greeted him. To help him engage in longer interactions, we practiced having him add a question in his response to a greeting. For example, he practiced saying, "Hi, how was your weekend?"; "Hi Jean, how's it going?"; or "Hey, how are you?" and then pausing for a response. Bill reported that adding a question after his greeting resulted in coworkers engaging in longer conversations with him, which boosted his confidence.

Compliments

Everyone enjoys compliments, but language samples of individuals on the autism spectrum show that compliments may be rare or nonexistent. Several studies have demonstrated that complimenting during sports and other activities can be improved through various methods, such as video modeling, modeling and prompting, practice, self-management, explicit rules, and social stories. Some studies show that teaching compliments generalizes to natural settings with new play or conversational partners (Almutlaq and Martella 2018; Apple et al. 2005; Macpherson et al. 2015). Individuals whose conversations lack compliments can be prompted to compliment people during games for good moves or winning. For some, this is difficult and needs to be explicitly prompted and practiced. In addition, we frequently teach our autistic individuals to cheer on others during team sports. For example, children sometimes do not want to participate in team activities or sports. In these instances, we give them the choice of either playing with the team or cheering on the team. Again, the wording of appropriate and sincere compliments and even cheering at the right times may need to be explicitly taught.

For adolescents and adults, an easy way to teach the initiation of compliments is to have the individual look for something different or new that the other person is wearing and then comment on that. For example, they can be prompted to say, "Those are pretty earrings," "Your necklace is beautiful," "Is that a new ring? It's pretty," or "Your hair looks nice. Did you get it cut?" For more general areas, we often have our patients tell us something they like about school, their parents, their siblings, and so on. If they respond with "I like it when my mom lets me play video games," we help them develop a compliment that is more appropriately related to the other person, such as "I appreciate when my mom gives me a ride to school" or "I like it when my brother plays Uno with me" or "Mom, I really like it when you help me with my homework." Practicing compliments can help the individual learn to use communication in a way that boosts another person's confidence. For many patients, it also can help them look at the glass as "half full" or come up with positives for a given situation.

Compliments should be both sincere and delivered in an authentic way. Giving too many at once, using a compliment to talk about oneself or manipulate another person, or giving the same compliment over and over again can seem insincere. When encouraging and prompting compliments, it is important to support the individual in learning to deliver them appropriately and with sincerity.

Case Example: Joaquin

> Joaquin, an autistic adult, lived at home with his single mother. He required quite a bit of supervision for daily living skills and routines, social support, and correct use of the internet. He frequently got mad at his mother when she attempted to help him or when she restricted his internet access after he visited inappropriate sites or posted inappropriate messages. Therefore, during our sessions we discussed compliments that he could give his mother. He was able to develop five sincere compliments, and when we read these to his mother, she started crying and said, "I never knew he appreciated the things I do for him." Thereafter, we practiced having him give regular compliments to others with whom he interacted. He reported that not only did this make the other person feel good but that he also felt good when he complimented others.

Conversing While Eating

Keeping a good conversation going during meals and snack times can be helpful for forming and maintaining relationships. School lunch tables provide nice opportunities for young children to mingle and chat. Observations during lunch periods at elementary schools show that many children discuss food while they are eating, which makes prompting easy for autistic children, who often show strengths in the visual area. Questions such as what peers have in their lunch, what foods they like and dislike, how they like the cafeteria foods served that day, what they like to drink, what their favorite dessert is, and so on are common conversation topics at the lunch table and can be prompted. In some situations, such as preschools, snacks can be arranged so that the children must ask each other for food and drink, such as saying, "Please pass the juice"; "Can I please have more crackers?"; or simply "juice" or "crackers" for children with less language. These social interactions have the benefit of resulting in natural reinforcers and encouraging peer social communication. For children who are more verbal, longer utterances can be prompted, such as asking "How many crackers do you want?"; "How much juice do you want?"; or "What's your favorite snack?"

For older elementary school–aged children and beyond (through adulthood), we encourage social conversation while eating. Prompting individuals to engage in social conversation between bites can be helpful. This can also help slow down eating for those who need it. Specifically, after each bite, we encourage the individual to put down the fork or food item, swallow the food, and answer a question, ask a question, or make a comment. Practice between bites can help the person get into a routine of social conversation during meals. Following the structured practice, the individual may not continue conversing after every bite, but it greatly improves socialization during meals.

Case Example: Shawn

Shawn, a college student, enjoyed dating but was concerned that although he had been on many first dates, very few women accepted a second date. During a conversation sample, it was observed that the bulk of his conversation during meals centered around his own interests and classes, he ate quickly and talked while eating, and he rarely appeared to take an interest in the conversational partner. In addition to working on slowing down and asking questions between bites, we practiced giving simple compliments relating to the other person's jewelry, clothes, and personality traits. Examples included "Those are pretty earrings, are they new?"; "That's a nice color on you"; and "Your trips are so interesting. Thanks for telling me about your vacation to Hawai'i." Including these additional functions of communication that showed his interest in another person made a difference in Shawn's dating life; soon after, he began a long-term relationship with another student.

Artificial Intelligence

Our team is also implementing artificial intelligence (AI) interventions for social communication to assist autistic adolescents and adults. Our research is showing that large language models can be used to provide live, actionable improvements in the social conversation of verbal autistic adolescents and adults that generalize to social conversation (L.K. Koegel et al. 2025). These types of computerized conversational agents may provide a more controlled and less socially demanding forum, which is often preferable for autistic individuals over face-to-face interventions, and may provide accessibility to individuals who lack trained providers or are awaiting services.

Summary

Social conversation is key to making friends, securing and maintaining employment, and developing interpersonal relationships, and differences or limitations can lead to a poorer quality of life. This area can be improved with practice for those who desire it. Treatments are available beginning in the preschool years and beyond. Preference and choice should be included whenever possible and implemented with peers in natural settings from very early on. Appropriate assessment and subsequent treatment to address challenging areas can improve social conversation, boost confidence, decrease co-occurring conditions, and raise overall pragmatic ratings as judged by others. Schools can be instrumental in addressing social conversation for those who could benefit from support in this area. Given that social conversation challenges tend to persist through the lifespan, even with highly verbal individuals, concentrated attention and continued support in this area are needed.

References

Almutlaq H, Martella RC: Teaching elementary-aged students with autism spectrum disorder to give compliments using a social story delivered through an iPad application. Int J Spec Educ 33(2):482–492, 2018

American Psychiatric Association: Diagnostic and Statistical Manual of Mental Disorders, 5th Edition, Text Revision. Washington, DC, American Psychiatric Association, 2022

Apple AL, Billingsley F, Schwartz IS, et al: Effects of video modeling alone and with self-management on compliment-giving behaviors of children with high-functioning ASD. J Posit Behav Interv 7(1):33–46, 2005

Chang YC, Dean M: Friendship interventions and measurements in children with ASD: a systematic review. Res Autism Spectr Disord 93:101947, 2022

Cremone IM, Carpita B, Nardi B, et al: Measuring social camouflaging in individuals with high functioning autism: a literature review. Brain Sci 13(3):469, 2023 36979279

Doggett RA, Krasno AM, Koegel LK, et al: Acquisition of multiple questions in the context of social conversation in children with autism. J Autism Dev Disord 43(9):2015–2025, 2013 23292139

Forrest DL, Kroeger RA, Stroope S: Autism spectrum disorder symptoms and bullying victimization among children with autism in the United States. J Autism Dev Disord 50(2):560–571, 2020 31691063

Hymas R, Badcock JC, Milne E: Loneliness in autism and its association with anxiety and depression: a systematic review with meta-analyses. Rev J Autism Dev Disord 11:121–156, 2022

Koegel LK, Park MN, Koegel RL: Using self-management to improve the reciprocal social conversation of children with autism spectrum disorder. J Autism Dev Disord 44(5):1055–1063, 2014 24127164

Koegel LK, Ashbaugh K, Navab A, et al: Improving empathic communication skills in adults with autism spectrum disorder. J Autism Dev Disord 46(3):921–933, 2016a 26520148

Koegel LK, Navab A, Ashbaugh K, et al: Using reframing to reduce negative statements in social conversation for adults with autism spectrum disorder. J Posit Behav Interv 18(3):133–144, 2016b

Koegel LK, Koplen Z, Koegel B, et al: Using a question bank intervention to improve socially initiated questions in adolescents and adults with autism. J Speech Lang Hear Res 64(4):1331–1339, 2021 33820435

Koegel LK, Ponder E, Bruzzese T, et al: Using artificial intelligence to improve empathetic statements in autistic adolescents and adults: a randomized clinical trial. J Autism Dev Disord 2025 [Epub ahead of print]

Macpherson K, Charlop MH, Miltenberger CA: Using portable video modeling technology to increase the compliment behaviors of children with autism during athletic group play. J Autism Dev Disord 45(12):3836–3845, 2015 24573335

9

Prognosis, Collateral Gains, and Strengths

Prognosis

When a child is diagnosed with autism spectrum disorder (ASD), parents want to understand their prognosis. Searching the internet can be depressing and unhelpful. Life expectancies are shorter for individuals on the spectrum, typically because of accidents (mostly drowning). Health issues are common; no pharmacological "cures" for ASD exist; and independent living and employment rates are low. However, it is important to bring parents' and providers' attention to the wider range of individuals being diagnosed with ASD, the greater emphasis on earlier diagnosis and intervention, and increased research in the area as reasons for optimism. Psychiatrists and providers can now make recommendations to parents that may lead to an improved prognosis.

Incoming Skills

The level of a child's skills when they enter treatment has been associated with improved outcomes following intervention programs. Children with higher language or cognitive skills are likely to make greater gains during intervention. One area that has been discussed extensively is the presence of verbal spoken communication. If intervention begins before age 3, 90%–95% of children can learn to use verbal communication; this drops slightly to 80%–85% if intervention begins after age 3 but drops dramatically to 20% if the child is still completely nonverbal at age 5 (L.K. Koegel 2000; R.L. Koegel et al. 2009). It is much more difficult to teach verbal spoken communication to children 5 years of age and older who are completely nonverbal. Thus, intervention for teaching expressive verbal communication is essential at the earliest possible time.

In addition to communication, IQ has been discussed in the literature as a prognostic indicator. It has been reported that about one-third to one-half (depending on the study) of children diagnosed with autism will test as having an intellectual disability (Autism and Developmental Disabilities Monitoring Network Surveillance Year 2008 Principal Investigators and Centers for Disease Control and Prevention 2012; Shenouda et al. 2023). Although it is unclear whether low IQ is a secondary effect of autism or vice versa, having a low IQ in early childhood appears to be associated with more characteristics of ASD (Denisova and Lin 2023).

Standardized Testing

There are several issues that families should understand when testing requires a behavioral response from the child. First, children on the autism spectrum are difficult to test, and standardized testing often underestimates their true functioning. This is the case for both cognitive and language tests. We conducted a study with preschool- and elementary school–aged autistic children with various interfering behaviors that appeared to impede their responsiveness on standardized tests. In this study, we functionally determined the behaviors that were interfering with test-taking and implemented individualized procedures to improve responsiveness (L.K. Koegel et al. 1997). The following are some examples.

Case Example: Donnie

> Donnie enjoyed looking at some of the standardized test items, but after an instruction such as "Point to the boy who is pushing the girl," he pointed to and named pictures that were irrelevant to the instruction or talked about items outside the window or around the room. Not attending or attending to irrelevant stimuli resulted in extremely low standardized test scores. Hypothesizing that this was an attention problem, we had him repeat the instruction: "Can you say, 'The boy is pushing the girl'?" Once he repeated the instruction, we would say, "Now point to it." This small manipulation resulted in significantly improved scores on his language and IQ tests.

Case Example: Brooks

> Brooks talked incessantly about cartoon characters, which interfered with his responsiveness on tests and led to extremely low standardized test scores, sometimes in the profoundly disabled range. Using this preferred interest, we offered him frequent breaks to discuss cartoon characters following a designated number of effortful responses to test questions. This resulted in greatly improved scores, with some in the average range.

Case Example: Coco

> Coco exhibited meltdowns, including tantrums and aggression, when asked to sit at a table with testing materials. However, these behaviors were not displayed when her mother was present. To improve her test scores, her mother sat silently in the room, only interacting to remind her to respond to the examiner. Coco attained completely different test results when her mother was present, with her scores moving from the profound to the average range when the testing situation was altered.

Although these manipulations slightly interfere with the standardization of the test, the question that arises relates to whether standardized testing is assessing behavior or true knowledge for a child on the autism spectrum. If a child scores low on a test but has acquired the knowledge, then placement, goals, and interventions may be developed that do not advance learning. Testing manipulations should not vary from the proper administration of test questions but should address the behaviors that may interfere with test-taking. For example, if a question is only supposed to be asked once, but the child is not attending, having the child repeat the question would not compromise administration of the test, whereas having the administrator repeat the question would. If standardized tests are given, and the child generally performs poorly on tests, the following questions can be asked:

- Does the child respond well in this setting? Some children respond better in a more comfortable setting rather than at a desk.
- Will the examiner bring out the best in the child? Many children respond better with a particular individual present or a particular tester who knows them.
- Is the test sensitive enough to provide useful, important, and practical information?
- Is the child's behavior likely to interfere with the testing, resulting in inaccurate outcomes?
- Is the child able to attend to the test instructions?

Another important issue for parents to understand is that sometimes test results, such as IQ, can change over time and may not be as meaningful as other measures, including adaptive functioning and communication (Solomon et al. 2023). Younger children on the autism spectrum can have more difficulties taking standardized tests, and children who have more skills and better communication early on may perform better on a standardized test (Solomon et al. 2023).

Also important is matching tests with the person who will be tested. If IQ testing is warranted, children with communication difficulties are likely to score higher on a nonverbal IQ test (Grondhuis et al. 2018). Furthermore, some standardized tests will not reflect the progress made by children with more significant impairments. For example, a 4-year-old child who has learned to use 5 consistent expressive verbal words and increases that number to 20 words following a month of targeted pivotal response treatment (PRT) intervention may still score within or below the lowest percentile on a standardized test, but this increase in verbalization is still a huge accomplishment for the child. Therefore, individualized probes, word inventories, language samples, functional observations, and clinician-made tests may be far more useful for monitoring a child's progress and for interpreting and understanding current functioning levels. Many schools will allow this type of testing in place of standardized tests because it can be more useful for developing goals and tracking progress.

Focus on Strengths

Low test scores for a child can be devastating to a parent. Although some children perform consistently throughout their lifespan, others do not, particularly those who have interfering behaviors and limited communication. Providers should help parents understand the limitations of standardized tests and perform a comprehensive evaluation of the child that also lists their strengths. Often, an individualized assessment that relies on observations is more informative and helpful. Parents need help understanding that testing may not tap into the strengths of their child, particularly if that child has restricted interests. Accumulating a vast amount of knowledge in a specific area may be instrumental in securing employment in later years, but this is unlikely to be reflected on a standardized test. Depression is extremely high among parents of children with autism and can negatively affect parenting. Making strengths-based assessments and focusing on the child's strengths during intervention can help decrease parental stress (Cosden et al. 2006; Steiner 2011; Steiner et al. 2012).

Prognosis

Although language and cognitive scores may be predictive of larger gains during short-term intervention studies, it is important to evaluate the child using a comprehensive battery that includes observations of language and behavior in natural settings in order to get a full and accurate picture of their functioning. Composite scores that consider a variety of areas (e.g., communication, daily living skills, socialization, motor skills, and behavior) can be helpful for predicting prognosis. The presence of language before age 5 is important (L.K. Koegel et al. 1999), so a focus on expressive communication at the earliest age possible is critical. Many consider autism to be a "lifelong disability," but research has shown that some children diagnosed with autism make incredible progress, and most clinics have documented cases of children making such large gains after intervention that they no longer qualify for the diagnosis (Sevin et al. 2024).

Case Example: My Nephew

My nephew's case is an example of tremendous progress. At age 2½, he had no consistent words and considerable interfering behaviors, including meltdowns, refusing to share toys, repetitively throwing objects, and screaming if anyone touched him, among other things. However, he had many strengths as well, including the ability to line up items in a specific organized order and focus intently on specific toys, and he quickly put together games and puzzles. He also inconsistently produced perfectly articulated words in appropriate contexts. After 3½ years of intensive PRT throughout his waking hours (this included intervention at family parties, when he was prompted to communicate and play with his cousins), he began to use spoken words; learned to share toys, take turns, and play with others; and began to excel at academics. He attended an inclusive preschool with two autistic children per class (the remaining students had no diagnosis).

We delayed starting kindergarten for a year to focus on his play with other children, and when he entered kindergarten, we decided not to send him with a "label." Although his kindergarten teacher was concerned about his frequent meltdowns, she described this as a typical part of child development, and they were addressed as such (e.g., using an earlier bedtime, prompted word use). We also focused on peer social interaction during lunch and daily after-school programs because he had some challenges taking turns, losing, and socializing with others. By the end of kindergarten, with this intensive support, he rarely had challenges with socialization. He now is a kind, compassionate, friendly, funny, and intelligent college student with lots of friends.

Many of the children with whom we have worked have gone to college, secured jobs, and married. Unfortunately, not all children have such positive outcomes, and for this reason, more intervention research is greatly needed. However, some important variables are known to lead to better outcomes; these are discussed in the sections that follow.

Collateral Gains

The goal of PRT is to accelerate the learning process. Autistic children have many challenges that need intervention; therefore, treatments that focus on widespread goals and, when targeted, will result in positive improvements in untreated behaviors are critical. When one is considering long-term outcomes, it is important to directly target areas that have added value and behaviors that will lead to *collateral gains*. Simply put, some things are more important to teach than others, and some target areas and implementation procedures have a broader impact than others. Originally, the PRT motivational procedures were developed because the children we were seeing in our clinic did not appear to enjoy sessions in which traditional applied behavior analysis (ABA) procedures were being implemented and would engage in avoidance behaviors and try to escape the sessions. Even children who engaged without interfering behaviors did not seem to enjoy the sessions; they did not seem particularly happy, interested, or enthusiastic.

Many newer "naturalistic" interventions incorporate the same variables described in our initial 1987 publication entitled "A Natural Language Teaching Paradigm for Nonverbal Autistic Children" (R.L. Koegel et al. 1987). These variables included a package of procedures designed to improve motivation. Each procedure had been previously researched in our clinics, and all were combined for this study. We eliminated the physical prompts that were commonly used to evoke correct articulation or sounds in nonverbal and minimally verbal children. Simply repeating the word was just as effective, and the physical prompting—such as gently pinching the child's lips together to prompt a bilabial sound—often annoyed the children and was not effective in improving articulation. Variables also included child choice in place of adult-chosen activities; we used age-appropriate items and activities that the children were likely to encounter in everyday settings, rather than the flash cards that were commonly used at that time. This led to more playful interactions than were possible with flash cards. For example, rolling a ball down a favorite ramp toy after saying "go" was fun for the child, and the adult could easily catch the ball at the bottom of the ramp to provide an additional opportunity for the child.

Along with more playful interactions, using child-preferred items and activities provides an opportunity for natural rewards rather than arbitrary (usually food) rewards. Although we encourage opportunities during meals and with snacks, foods are used in the context of the teaching activity rather than as an arbitrary reward for a correct response. For example, if the child requests the food item, it is provided as a natural reward for responding. Likewise, during academic instruction, if the child is asked to write a letter, word, or sentence about a food item or to add food items during a math activity, that food item is provided as a natural reward. Our research also led us to understand that rewarding all true attempts results in better responding than a stricter shaping model that rewards only responses that are better than the previous response. These strategies, although sometimes renamed over the years, provide the foundation for most naturalistic interventions described today, and when incorporated, they result in improved motivation and collateral gains.

When and Where?

With any child, frequent opportunities for learning are critical, and they may be even more important for children on the autism spectrum because most of these children do not initiate interactions spontaneously. Many parents ask how many hours per day of intervention is optimal, and the answer is "all of their waking hours." However, our recommendations do not require parents to sit their children down and drill them repeatedly. Potential opportunities arise frequently throughout the day in all natural settings. For example, if a child who is learning first words enjoys going for car rides, the parent can prompt the word "car" before getting in the car for a ride. Gradually, more words can be included. For example, the parents can prompt "open" to open the house door, "key" while taking out a key, "car" while getting in the car, "buckle" while seat-belting the child, "go" when driving, and so on. These activities then lead to the natural reward of the enjoyable drive. For some children, prompts such as "stop" and "go" can be provided in the car at stop signs and stop lights. After arriving at the grocery store, favorite items can be selected, and the child can be prompted to say words related to desired grocery items, such as "cracker" and "more." The same routine can be implemented when returning home. Although this requires ongoing effort on the parents' and providers' parts, practicing social communication throughout the day in all settings will lead to greater communicative gains. Coordination and parent education are important for a seamless program.

How?

Fidelity of implementation (FoI) is important. FoI means that intervention procedures are being used in the same manner as were described in the published study. Most unsuccessful programs fail because they are not implemented properly, not because the procedures are ineffective. Many studies are implemented by highly educated and extremely experienced researchers. However, in everyday life, these programs may be implemented by less skilled staff members or parents who are busy with other children, work, and household tasks. One preschooler was not rewarded for his first word, "push," when he approached a teacher requesting to be pushed on the swing because the teacher was "taking a break." I often tell parents that if their child requires a lot of prompting to respond, and they are in a hurry, it is better to not start a teaching opportunity at that moment. If the parent is not consistent, children will not get the connection between the prompt and the need to respond. Instead, they may learn that not responding is the desired behavior.

The most successful programs require parents to actively participate, and it is important to provide "practice with feedback," wherein a parent or provider is observed implementing the intervention and given feedback on areas that are not being administered properly. For PRT, we score each area so the parent or professional is given specific feedback on their implementation. We have parents work with their child for 10 minutes while we score each minute according to the FoI sheet and the directions provided in the appendix to this chapter. Parents and providers must score 80% or higher to pass our FoI assessment because implementing the intervention as developed and intended is critical for an optimal child outcome.

Response to Intervention

Response to intervention or *response to treatment* refers to whether the intervention is effective in creating the desired change in the targeted area. As with any behavioral, communicative, social, or academic program, progress must be measured in an unbiased and systematic way. This usually involves observing and tallying behaviors. An appropriate evaluation system should be in place for each area targeted. Some areas benefit from frequent monitoring, such as when a child is first beginning to use words and coordination is important, or when a child is aggressive or engaging in behaviors that interfere with family or classroom functioning. Other behaviors do not need daily monitoring, and recording data too frequently can interfere with the flow of instruction and teaching time. Many programs are available for targeting given areas, but these programs sometimes need to be adjusted or replaced if they are not yielding the intended effects. Monitoring will indicate whether a program is effective or a change is warranted. Some children will show change in one setting but not in others, so understanding the context of these settings can be helpful when determining if change is needed.

Coordination

Coordination of programs is also imperative for individuals with autism. Behavioral contrast, in which contingencies vary from one setting to another, can cause an increase in unwanted behaviors. For example, if a child whines and cries and is rewarded by being picked up in one setting but is required to use the word "up" in another setting, the use of the whining is more likely to increase than the use of the word. This can also occur with punishment; if a child is punished at home for grabbing toys from siblings but is not punished for grabbing toys from peers at school, the grabbing at home may decrease, but the grabbing at school may increase. Sometimes we also see carryover effects from different contingencies in different settings.

Case Example: Coordinating Goals

> Divorced parents had different bedtime routines. At one home, the child read three stories in bed before the light was turned off. He developed great sleeping habits in this setting. In contrast, the other parent succumbed to demands for a cup of water, another story, a stroller ride, and so on, which made bedtime a problem, with little sleep happening in that setting. After the transition back to the other parent, it took a few days of addressing the interfering behaviors to get back into the productive bedtime routine. Once the parents coordinated with the three-story routine, however, the child's sleep patterns greatly improved, which made life easier for both parents.

Without coordination of goals and intervention methods, progress may be slow or nonexistent. In some cases, increases in unwanted behaviors may result. Therefore, having everyone on the same page—which may involve compromises by all parties—will lead to the best outcomes for the child.

Who Is Providing the Intervention?

For many school and in-home intervention programs, the individual spending the most direct hours with the child often has the least professional training. For this reason, it is important for parents to express themselves if something does not feel right. Several important variables should be considered. First is the importance of the target goals. Often, school personnel who are with the child are not aware of the target goals. With your help, parents may want to draft a "cheat sheet" that describes simplified target goals and facts about the child. An example of this is shown in Figure 9.1. A second issue is fidelity. Once parents have received training and understand FoI, they can coordinate

---

Behavior Cheat Sheet

If David is out of his seat or off-task for 5 seconds...give him a prompt!

1. Reminders to stay on-task (with peers whenever possible!)

PEER STRATEGIES

  a. Peer (prompt peer): Have a peer buddy remind him to line up/transition/find the assignment. "Sally, can you remind David where to put that paper?"

  b. Peer: Have him ask a friend what the assignment is.

TEACHER STRATEGIES

  c. Teacher prompt: Peer – "What are your friends doing?" "Look at Sally, what is she doing?"

  d. Teacher: "What did Mr. Brown ask you to do?" "Listen to Mr. Brown...he is giving directions now."

  e. Nonverbal: Tap shoulder and point to teacher if he isn't listening in lesson.

  f. Nonverbal: Point to cubby if he needs to get a folder from cubby, point to line if he is supposed to be lining up, etc.

  g. General: "What was the direction?"

  h. General: "Who can you ask if you do not know?"

2. Giving choices

  a. "Do you want to write with a regular pencil or a colored pencil?" (to help him get started)

  b. "Do you want me to highlight where the words should go, or do you want to write without it?" (offer some help but don't do the work for him)

  c. "Do you want to write two sentences or three sentences today?" (give him two choices where he is still doing an appropriate amount of work but has some control over how much)

  d. "Do you want to play Legos for 15 more seconds or 20 more seconds?" (only use if he is having a hard time transitioning away from the activity)

  e. "Do you want to play the math game once and earn reward time, or play twice?" (we probably know the answer to this, but it gives him some choice and motivates him to play for that reward)

  f. "Do you want to earn time with Legos or putty?"

3. Reward systems (it helps to know what David is motivated by at that moment!)

  a. Free choice time: "When you finish this, you can get 2 minutes of playing with putty!"

  b. Reward with more preferred activity (using what he wants to do in that moment): "You want to read *Princess Candy*? Great idea! You can definitely read it right after we read two chapters of the assigned book!"

  c. Positive reinforcement: "Wow, you are doing such a good job, I can't wait for (Mr. Peschl) or (Mom) to see your work!" **Consider creating a checklist for good behavior that he takes home each day.**

  d. Positive language: Instead of "We can't play on the iPad right now," say, "You bet we can do that as soon as we finish our math game!" (keeps the language positive and turns it into a motivation!)

4. Clear away distractions

  a. If playing with iPad during lesson instead of listening, quietly take iPad to hold (not punishment, just holding on to it until he needs it).

  b. Drawing on dry-erase board during math lesson when he should be looking at smartboard? Hand him marker when he needs it, hold it when he doesn't.

5. Redirection

  a. Trying to play with projector/smartboard? Redirect his attention: "Oh, I see a good open spot by Sally to stand for GoNoodle!"

  b. Crawling under the table during math game? Try saying "Uh-oh, your partner almost rolled the dice right off the table!" "Let's see how fast you can get that finished."

Figure 9.1 Behavior cheat sheet.

and provide specific direct feedback or make suggestions to a supervisor, who then can provide additional training. For example, one family noticed that their provider only worked on maintenance tasks, and their child was not progressing. Once the supervisor was made aware of this and gave specific feedback, the child began making progress. Providers must be aware of goals and implement them frequently. One child's in-home program had social goals to be prompted with neighborhood children. However, the provider did not like going outside, so no social goals were implemented. Once the parents reported this to the company, the child was assigned a new provider who enjoyed being outside and could prompt the goals.

Again, it is helpful to have parents keep an eye open and assess other providers on proper and frequent implementation of treatment. Many programs and schools do not have adequate training or provide supervision of aides and technicians. All too often, children on the autism spectrum can be seen pacing the perimeter of the playground, when this valuable time could be used to prompt social behavior. Some paraprofessionals will stand back and watch, intervening only if the child is getting into trouble. Proper training and frequent supervision are helpful. Data collection by the individuals spending the most time with the child can also be helpful for ensuring goals are being implemented and the child is progressing.

Figure 9.1 is an example "cheat sheet" for an elementary school–aged student who was fully included in general education. These types of supplemental materials can be helpful for coordinating across providers.

How Much Intervention?

Parents often ask how much intervention a child needs. Intervention needs to be implemented throughout all the child's waking hours. This may be a combination of support from school, in-home programs, and time with parents and others, but, for best results, programs should be consistent across all settings and times. Some children also will need programs implemented at night if they have sleep difficulties. Along with the notion of constant and consistent intervention is the importance of providing enough opportunities for learning. Our PRT FoI requires that individuals provide at least two opportunities per minute. Although this is not possible during all of a child's waking hours, providing an adequate number of learning opportunities across all settings is important. Too often, children on the autism spectrum spend hours alone, with excessive screen time or otherwise unengaged. As with any child, providing an ongoing therapeutic environment can lead to better outcomes. Children acquire target areas more rapidly if the program is consistent and implemented frequently across all settings.

Carefully Picking Goals

There are essential considerations when developing goals. First and foremost, the goals should be meaningful. Ask if the goal will be helpful in both the short and long run. Goals should address the challenges accompanying the core characteristics of autism that interfere with everyday life and independence, such as social communication, self-help, engagement, academics, and behavior. Most autistic individuals do not have a regular vigorous exercise program built into their routines, but these have been shown to be effective for focus, fitness, weight, and health and can lead to social interaction opportunities. Thus, physical activity should always be a goal (Lang et al. 2010). Other areas appear to provide added value for the child. For example, teaching question-asking helps with long-term outcomes (L.K. Koegel et al. 1999). Exposing children to a variety of verbs (Crandall et al. 2019), recasting their utterances with slightly longer utterances, and, whenever possible, having them repeat the longer utterances seem to help them develop. It is also important that adults not simplify the linguistic input too much or model incorrect grammar (e.g., deleting articles and other words that do not affect the semantic intent) as the child's language develops.

For many parents, it is helpful to remember SMART—Specific, Measurable, Achievable, Relevant, Timebound—goals. A goal should be specifically stated. For example, if a child's goal is to learn vocabulary words, the specific words to learn should be stated so that all involved can target this area. If a goal is for the child to learn to read, the number of words per minute, accuracy, and level and type of comprehension being measured should be stated. Once goals are articulated in the child's individualized education program (IEP) or home plan, we recommend adding details about how and how often they should be measured and when the child is expected to complete each goal. An individual's goals should be realistic and attainable in order to decrease frustration, but they should offer enough of a reach to help the individual function at an optimal level.

Collateral Gains Offered by New Interventions

PRT and other naturalistic interventions consider the child's motivation by using child choice, natural rewards, and other variables to improve responsiveness and engagement. Individuals who are enjoying learning and social communication are more likely to frequently and eagerly engage, which is critical for this population. When incorporating the

PRT motivational components, we see greater collateral gains in areas such as joint attention (Ebrahim 2019; Vismara and Lyons 2007), pragmatics, socialization, nonverbal pragmatic areas (Mohammadzaheri et al. 2014), interfering and disruptive behaviors (R.L. Koegel et al. 1992), and overall affect, including interest, happiness, and engagement (Dunlap 1984). Given the central goal of accelerating the learning process for these children, target areas and general procedures that lead to collateral gains are especially crucial.

Skill or Performance Deficit

Individuals on the autism spectrum often have difficulty generalizing newly learned behaviors to new settings or with different people. While developing goals, it can be helpful to assess whether the individual is demonstrating a skill deficit or a performance deficit. A *skill deficit* refers to a particular behavior that the individual has not yet learned. A *performance deficit* refers to a behavior that the individual has acquired but is not using appropriately in all settings. These deficits require different interventions, so to make the best use of valuable and limited time, it is important to ensure the team understands goals that have not been acquired (skill) versus behaviors that simply need prompting in natural environments (performance).

Inclusion

Inclusion, in which all children, regardless of differences, are educated together, is a philosophical concept that most people embrace. It can reduce stigma, provide equal and similar opportunities for all, and benefit all students when teachers learn to individualize instruction. Children with disabilities are entitled to an education in the least restrictive environment, meaning that children with autism are entitled to be educated in a general education classroom with similarly aged peers. *Full inclusion* means that a child with disabilities has been placed in general education throughout the day, with no assignment to a special education classroom. *Partial inclusion* means that a child with disabilities spends part of their day in general education and part of their day in a specialized setting.

Inclusion offers many benefits. For students with autism, inclusive settings have been shown to be superior for socialization (Dean and Chang 2021) and academic performance (Kurth and Mastergeorge 2010). However, and unfortunately, many teachers are ill-prepared to provide the accommodations necessary for inclusion, resulting in failed programs. Creating a supportive environment may necessitate creating an individualized curriculum, implementing social programs, encouraging peer support and peer education, increasing parent-teacher communication, and collaborating across all settings. Furthermore, positive attitudes toward inclusion by teachers and school administrators increase successful implementation (Russell et al. 2023). Simply placing a child in regular education without proper support is unlikely to be effective and may even be detrimental; however, properly implemented programs can result in widespread improvements that are often greater than those achieved by children placed in special education classrooms (Kurth and Mastergeorge 2010). Thus, proper preparation, program implementation, and support in inclusive school and community environments can greatly enhance a child's outcome.

Advocacy

Individuals on the autism spectrum frequently need others to advocate for them, especially when they have social communication challenges. Unfortunately, individuals with disabilities often experience various forms of discrimination. Support for their rights, welfare, and ability to secure services often requires oversight and persistence. Physicians and other professionals can support patients by encouraging parents to ask for a wide range of programs in school, home, and community settings. Educating the greater community, including classmates, school personnel, potential employers, and others, also leads to greater understanding and acceptance. Groups now exist for people with "profound autism" or high support needs that, among other things, advocate for research and services for this high-need population. For individuals who are highly verbal, self-advocacy can be helpful for independent living, employment, and socialization. Advocacy that focuses on the strengths of individuals with autism will have long-lasting positive effects. Autistic advocacy groups can be helpful as well in providing support for individuals with varying support needs.

Neurodiversity Movement

Another area that is important to discuss is the neurodiversity movement. In the late 1990s, sociologist Judy Singer discussed the notion of *neurodiversity* in her honors thesis, suggesting that disabilities may not necessarily be a medical condition but a natural and important part of humanity. Her reported personal experiences with autism led her to propose the idea that some individuals' brains simply work differently.

This idea has gained momentum, with discussions of both benefits and challenges to this movement. On the positive side, advocates have called for more education and acceptance from the general public, stating that many behaviors do not need intervention. For example, advocates suggest that some behaviors that provide comfort (e.g., repetitive behaviors) or discomfort (e.g., eye contact) for neurodiverse people should be considered a difference, rather than a problem, and that society should be more understanding of them. Some neurodiverse individuals report that early ABA procedures, which commonly used various, sometimes painful punishments, caused PTSD in individuals exposed to them. Some neurodiversity advocates suggest that no intervention whatsoever should be provided to individuals diagnosed with ASD. On the other hand, some parents of children more affected by ASD suggest that those in the neurodiverse movement who have the verbal and cognitive ability to opine should not attempt to represent those who are minimally verbal or nonverbal (also referred to as having profound autism). Similarly, many parents and neurodiverse and autistic individuals report that intervention has been helpful and should be continued. Fortunately, PRT and other naturalistic interventions that emerged following initial work in the 1970s and 1980s (R.L. Koegel et al. 1987; McGee et al. 1985) consider factors such as strengths-based principles, child choice, motivation, and natural consequences and can be particularly helpful in promoting communication, play, and social engagement. Rather than focusing on behavior reduction, PRT considers child motivation, as measured by affect scales of happiness, interest, enthusiasm, and general behavior, to be an important indicator during intervention sessions. Because of this, many researchers, including neurodiverse researchers, have endorsed PRT and similar interventions that consider these important components (Schuck et al. 2022).

Independent Living

Prognosis can be improved by ensuring that meaningful goals are selected to target. Independent living skills have been largely neglected in IEPs. Important areas for independent living include socialization and social communication, education and employment, vocational skills, self-help, and self-determination (Findley et al. 2022). The relationship between daily living skills and independent living necessitates programming that focuses on areas such as shopping, money management, hygiene, safety, laws, socialization, cooking, employment, and so on. Creating independence in these areas should begin early in a child's life, with a deeper focus during the transition to adulthood. Parents may need support in developing goals, with follow-through occurring in all settings. Independent living and community participation should be a possibility for most individuals on the autism spectrum, but careful planning across the lifespan is crucial to make this goal a reality.

Summary

Parents often ask their psychiatrists and providers about prognosis. Thoughtful discussion about how motivational a child's interventions are is important. When motivational components are included, the individual will be an active learner, as seen by their positive affect, engagement, and high responsivity. Implementing motivational procedures results in various collateral gains that accelerate the learning process. Taking an active role in parent education and choosing meaningful areas to tackle are also important for improved child gains. Parents have many decisions to make throughout their child's life. Collaborative and consistent efforts among providers and across settings will result in the greatest and fastest gains. Most importantly, the learning process should be enjoyable for the child, and this can be monitored by assessing their engagement and high affect during intervention sessions. Ensuring that the PRT components are incorporated throughout the day will improve affect, engagement, and learning.

References

Autism and Developmental Disabilities Monitoring Network Surveillance Year 2008 Principal Investigators, Centers for Disease Control and Prevention: Prevalence of autism spectrum disorders—Autism and Developmental Disabilities Monitoring Network, 14 sites, United States, 2008. MMWR Surveill Summ 61(3):1–19, 2012 22456193

Cosden M, Koegel LK, Koegel RL, et al: Strength-based assessment for children with autism spectrum disorders. Res Pract Persons Severe Disabil 31(2):134–143, 2006

Crandall MC, Bottema-Beutel K, McDaniel J, et al: Children with autism spectrum disorder may learn from caregiver verb input better in certain engagement states. J Autism Dev Disord 49(8):3102–3112, 2019 31073750

Dean M, Chang YC: A systematic review of school-based social skills interventions and observed social outcomes for students with autism spectrum disorder in inclusive settings. Autism 25(7):1828–1843, 2021 34231405

Denisova K, Lin Z: The importance of low IQ to early diagnosis of autism. Autism Res 16(1):122–142, 2023 36373182

Dunlap G: The influence of task variation and maintenance tasks on the learning and affect of autistic children. J Exp Child Psychol 37(1):41–64, 1984 6707578

Ebrahim MTES: Effectiveness of a pivotal response training programme in joint attention and social interaction of kindergarten children with autism spectrum disorder. Psycho-Educational Research Reviews 8(2):48–56, 2019

Findley JA, Ruble LA, McGrew JH: Individualized education program quality for transition age students with autism. Res Autism Spectr Disord 91:101900, 2022 35096138

Grondhuis SN, Lecavalier L, Arnold LE, et al: Differences in verbal and nonverbal IQ test scores in children with autism spectrum disorder. Res Autism Spectr Disord 49:47–55, 2018

Koegel LK: Interventions to facilitate communication in autism. J Autism Dev Disord 30(5):383–391, 2000 11098873

Koegel LK, Koegel RL, Smith A: Variables related to differences in standardized test outcomes for children with autism. J Autism Dev Disord 27(3):233–243, 1997 9229256

Koegel LK, Koegel RL, Shoshan Y, et al: Pivotal response intervention II: preliminary long-term outcome data. J Assoc Pers Sev Handicaps 24(3):186–198, 1999

Koegel RL, O'Dell MC, Koegel LK: A natural language teaching paradigm for nonverbal autistic children. J Autism Dev Disord 17(2):187–200, 1987 3610995

Koegel RL, Koegel LK, Surratt A: Language intervention and disruptive behavior in preschool children with autism. J Autism Dev Disord 22(2):141–153, 1992 1378049

Koegel RL, Shirotova L, Koegel LK: Antecedent stimulus control: using orienting cues to facilitate first-word acquisition for nonresponders with autism. Behav Anal 32(2):281–284, 2009 22478527

Kurth JA, Mastergeorge AM: Academic and cognitive profiles of students with autism: implications for classroom practice and placement. Int J Spec Educ 25(2):8–14, 2010

Lang R, Koegel LK, Ashbaugh K, et al: Physical exercise and individuals with autism spectrum disorders: a systematic review. Res Autism Spectr Disord 4(4):565–576, 2010

McGee GG, Krantz PJ, McClannahan LE: The facilitative effects of incidental teaching on preposition use by autistic children. J Appl Behav Anal 18(1):17–31, 1985 3997695

Mohammadzaheri F, Koegel LK, Rezaee M, et al: A randomized clinical trial comparison between pivotal response treatment (PRT) and structured applied behavior analysis (ABA) intervention for children with autism. J Autism Dev Disord 44(11):2769–2777, 2014 24840596

Russell A, Scriney A, Smyth S: Educator attitudes towards the inclusion of students with autism spectrum disorders in mainstream education: a systematic review. Rev J Autism Dev Disord 10:477–491, 2023

Schuck RK, Tagavi DM, Baiden KMP, et al: Neurodiversity and autism intervention: reconciling perspectives through a naturalistic developmental behavioral intervention framework. J Autism Dev Disord 52(10):4625–4645, 2022 34643863

Sevin IE, Dogan N, Ozbaran NB: Characteristics of individuals losing autism diagnosis: a comparative study with typically developing and autism spectrum disorder individuals. Early Interv Psychiatry 19(1):e13617, 2024 39435879

Shenouda J, Barrett E, Davidow AL, et al: Prevalence and disparities in the detection of autism without intellectual disability. Pediatrics 151(2):e2022056594, 2023 36700335

Solomon M, Cho B, Iosif AM, et al: IQ trajectories in autistic children through preadolescence. JCPP Adv 3(1):e12127, 2023 37397281

Steiner AM: A strength-based approach to parent education for children with autism. J Posit Behav Interv 13(3):178–190, 2011

Steiner AM, Koegel LK, Koegel RL, et al: Issues and theoretical constructs regarding parent education for autism spectrum disorders. J Autism Dev Disord 42(6):1218–1227, 2012 21336525

Vismara LA, Lyons GL: Using perseverative interests to elicit joint attention behaviors in young children with autism: theoretical and clinical implications for understanding motivation. J Posit Behav Interv 9(4):214–228, 2007

Chapter Appendix: Pivotal Response Treatment Fidelity of Implementation

Pivotal Response Treatment (PRT) Fidelity of Implementation Assessment Form

Motivational Procedures for Teaching Beginning Verbal Social-Communication

Name of Participant:		Date Scored:		Purpose:
Name of Child:		Scored By::		Title of Video:

Interval (1-min)	Child attending and appropriate and clear opportunities	Maintenance tasks and task variation	Child choice and follow lead	Shared Control	Contingent	Natural	Contingent on attempts	Notes
1								
2								
3								
4								
5								

Figure 9.2 Pivotal Response Treatment (PRT) Fidelity of Implementation Assessment Form (page 1).

6						
7						
8						
9						
10						
% Accurate Implementation of Component						

Global Categories:	Yes/No	Intervention implemented in the natural environment.	Additional Feedback Notes:
	Yes/No	Opportunities provided in the context of interactive play-based activities with the individual observed demonstrating high level of play involvement and positive affect.	
	Yes/No	Intervention is conducted with parent involvement (if applicable).	

Figure 9.3 Pivotal Response Treatment (PRT) Fidelity of Implementation Assessment Form (page 2).

Instructions

Fidelity of implementation (FoI) for pivotal response treatment (PRT) is scored across 10 intervals lasting 1 minute each.

An *opportunity for language* is defined as any directive, verbal model prompt, forced-choice opportunity, carrier phrase, closed-ended question, open-ended question, or time delay intentionally set up by the individual being observed that clearly indicates to the child that a specific verbal response directly related to the task, opportunity, and natural reinforcer is required. A new opportunity for language is recorded if the child produces a verbal response, or when at least 2 seconds elapse without a verbal response from the child and the adult re-presents the same (or similar) prompt, moves up the prompt hierarchy, or moves on to a new opportunity.

For Level II and III PRT training and certification, the individual being observed must provide at least two opportunities for the child to respond with expressive verbalizations within each 1-minute interval. Additionally, at least two opportunities within each interval must be tied to a tangible natural reinforcer (e.g., item or action directly related to the opportunity and child response, which the child receives as a functional consequence of their use of language), unless this is not appropriate to the developmental level of the child or to the teaching context. Accordingly, 1-minute time intervals that offer fewer than two opportunities for verbal communication directly tied to a tangible natural reinforcer are scored as incorrect (–) across all categories. The individual being observed must be actively seeking out opportunities.

Pause the video clip after each opportunity or 1-minute interval and score each of the PRT motivational components.

Score each component as

- **+ (plus):** The individual being observed used this component of PRT correctly across the *majority* of opportunities provided in the time interval.
- **– (minus):** The PRT component was not demonstrated by the individual being observed or was used incorrectly by the individual across the *majority* of opportunities in the time interval. A (–) is also recorded if no majority is established (e.g., 50% accurate implementation, 50% inaccurate implementation).
- **N/A (not applicable):** The child is not at an appropriate level for this PRT component (e.g., multiple cues), the scorer is not familiar with the child (e.g., to know which opportunities are maintenance tasks), the individual being observed did not have an opportunity to implement this PRT motivational component due to the teaching context, or the component is not appropriate/necessary for the interval.

Additional Scoring Instructions

If an opportunity is started during one 1-minute interval and carries over to the following interval, the opportunity is scored for the initial interval in which the opportunity was provided (i.e., the interval within which the opportunity started).

Intervals that have fewer than two opportunities tied to a natural reinforcer are scored as incorrect (–) in all categories. The individual being observed must be actively seeking out opportunities. The individual being observed is not penalized if they do not provide an opportunity/second opportunity within an interval because they are following through on a previously provided opportunity, waiting out an interfering behavior, attempting to actively engage the child with no success, and so on.

The performance of the individual being observed should be scored independently of the child's response.

Individuals being observed must score 80% (8 out of 10) or more in each category to meet FoI for PRT.

Definitions

Child Attending

The individual being observed must have the child's attention prior to presenting an opportunity. For example, the child's attention can be demonstrated by the child looking at the adult or in the adult's direction or at or in the direction of the motivating stimulus item(s) related to the opportunity for verbal communication. Additionally, it is important that the child is not overly distracted by the activity at hand. The adult should maintain the child's attention while presenting the opportunities.

Appropriate and Clear Opportunities

The opportunity (discriminative stimulus or S^D) for the child to respond must be *clear, uninterrupted* (by, e.g., repetitive or disruptive behavior), *and appropriate* to the activity, task, and natural reinforcer(s). The individual being observed should provide simple and straightforward opportunities, with limited extraneous language. Expectations for responding should be explicit, and there should be a direct and functional connection between the adult opportunity, the targeted (child) response, and the naturally reinforcing consequence of that response (i.e., obtaining the desired item or action corresponding to a request). Prompting procedures should be accurately implemented according to the PRT guidelines for teaching first words and multiple-word utterances, and the antecedents used should be appropriate to the developmental level of the child. Additionally, prompts should remain consistent when re-presenting a prompt within an opportunity (when a child does not respond to an initial prompt or responds with an incorrect or inappropriate response) unless the adult is moving up the prompt hierarchy. The prompt hierarchy must be used correctly if applicable. Finally, opportunities for verbal communication (prompts and target responses) must be developmentally appropriate and appropriate to the context.

Interspersing Maintenance Tasks/Task Variation

The individual being observed should intersperse *maintenance tasks* (i.e., tasks the child has already mastered and can perform with relative ease) with acquisition tasks (i.e., new and more challenging tasks that the child does not yet have in their repertoire). Maintenance tasks can be differentiated from acquisition tasks across several variables, including, for example, word (new word or learned word), length of utterance, and type of antecedent (e.g., response to verbal model prompt, forced-choice, carrier phrase, closed-ended question, open-ended question, time delay). Additionally, the individual should vary tasks across each activity. Specifically, each 1-minute interval must include a minimum of one instance of task variation and one maintenance task. This category should not be recorded unless the scorer is familiar with the child of the individual being observed and has been given a detailed outline of maintenance and acquisition tasks. If a child is at the very beginning stages of verbal communication acquisition, when they may not yet have many (or any) word attempts that are maintenance items (even in response to verbal model prompts), receptive language opportunities may also be scored as maintenance tasks.

Child Choice and Follow the Child's Lead

To a large extent, the individual being observed should *follow the child's lead* in selecting activities and stimulus materials and guiding the direction of the activity. The individual being observed should provide opportunities for the child to *make choices* within and across activities. Activities should be *child directed*. Using child choice can be objectively defined as 1) providing two or more alternatives for the child to choose from, for example, "Do you want to play with the bubbles or ride the bike?"; 2) allowing the child to accept or reject an offer, for example, "Do you want to swing?"; 3) prompting the child to respond to an open-ended question, for example, "What do you want?"; or 4) following the child's lead in selecting and/or directing activities by responding to the verbal or nonverbal initiations of choosing an activity, object, or action. For example, the child reaches for the Play-Doh and says, "Doh!" and the parent begins to incorporate Play-Doh into the interaction, or the child and adult are playing with cars, and the adult prompts "down" before the child is able to slide the car down the ramp. The child begins to move the cars up the ramp, so the parent follows this motivating interest and begins prompting "up." If the child is attempting to avoid the interaction or is not showing interest in the current task, the individual being observed should actively attempt to change the activity.

Shared Control

The individual being observed must have *shared control* of the activities and stimulus materials at all times, especially when given opportunities for verbal communication, so that natural opportunities with contingent reinforcement can be provided. This includes tangible shared control of stimuli as well as accurate use of interruption procedures as appropriate. The individual must also assume control should the child engage in hazardous (e.g., self-injurious) or inappropriate behavior. It also may be important for the individual being observed to have shared control not only of the stimulus materials related to the opportunity but also of anything that the child may be engaged in or attending to at the time the opportunity is provided.

Contingent

Reinforcement must be *contingent* on the child's behavior. The consequential response of the individual being observed (e.g., giving the child a toy) must be dependent on the child's response (e.g., the child saying "toy"). Once an opportunity has been provided, if the child does not make a correct verbal response or a good attempt to respond verbally, or if the child engages in inappropriate (e.g., disruptive) behavior, the adult should not provide the reinforcer. Reinforcement should be provided contingent (conditionally) on a response specific to the provided opportunity (e.g., if the adult provides a verbal model prompt for a two-word combination, the reinforcement should be contingent on a good imitative attempt at the two-word combination. If the adult asks what color block a child wants and the child responds, "Block," the reinforcing item should not be provided). If the child does not respond or responds with an incorrect or inappropriate response, the adult should re-present the initial prompt or move up the prompt hierarchy. If the adult has re-presented the opportunity (and moved up the prompt hierarchy) and the child still does not respond with a good attempt, loses interest in the natural reinforcer, or begins to become overly frustrated, the adult should simply put the reinforcer aside and move on to a new interaction, natural reinforcer, and opportunity.

Additionally, reinforcement must be provided *immediately* following the child's appropriate response or reasonable attempt. The response-to-reinforcer ratio should be kept at 1:1. Each time the child responds with a correct response or a reasonable attempt, the child should be rewarded with the tangible, naturally reinforcing consequence (e.g., item or action related to the request).

Natural

Reinforcement should be *directly related* to the activity/task and must be functionally related to the child's verbal response and a *natural consequence* of the target behavior. For example, the individual being observed should provide the child with the item requested or engage with the child in the requested activity or action, rather than provide a reward that is unrelated to the verbalization (e.g., providing a train after the child requests "train" instead of handing the child a piece of candy or star sticker). At least two opportunities within each 1-minute time interval must have a tangible natural reinforcer (e.g., object or action directly related to the child's response).

Contingent on Attempts

Any *goal-directed attempt* to respond to questions, instructions, or opportunities should be reinforced. Although an attempt does not necessarily need to be completely correct, it must be *reasonable*. A reasonable attempt is commonly demonstrated by attention to the task and a response that is directly related to the opportunity, shows clear intent to respond, and demonstrates clear effort. It is important that the individual being observed be consistent with what they consider a "good attempt" by the child (and what is or is not appropriate to reinforce) for a specific target behavior across an opportunity, interval, and activity.

There is a close connection between *contingent reinforcement, natural reinforcement*, and *being contingent on attempts*. Specifically, if the individual being observed does not remain contingent, the individual is also not rewarding correct responses or attempts, so this is no longer a natural consequence for the child's behavior. Due to this connection, when a "contingent" or "contingent on attempts" component is scored as (–), all three components (contingent, natural, and contingent on attempts) are typically scored (–).

10

Clinical Considerations

As I have discussed throughout this book, autism is a complex neurological condition with varying characteristics. Autistic individuals can range from completely nonverbal to highly verbal and may have restricted and repetitive behaviors that vary from accumulating a vast amount of information on a given subject to performing motor repetitions that can interfere with everyday engagement. However, regardless of needs, some important universal considerations should be taken into account.

Motivation

Motivation is the key to improving responsiveness and correct responding, as well as decreasing disruptive and interfering behaviors. Most programs that support autistic individuals now use naturalistic procedures that include choice and other important variables to improve participants' motivation. Pivotal response treatment (PRT) has carefully defined these variables, and parents and providers can be objectively scored on their implementation. When the PRT motivational variables are incorporated into an intervention, faster learning occurs, and the learner's affect is improved with regard to levels of happiness, enthusiasm, and interest. Individuals also make advances in communication style and other key untargeted areas. In addition, when parents learn to implement the motivational procedures, their affect in terms of happiness and interest also improves, and their stress decreases (R.L. Koegel et al. 1996). PRT has been shown to be effective in home, school, and community settings and with teachers, speech-language pathologists, parents, paraprofessionals, and other care providers as intervention agents when compared with treatment as usual or structured applied behavior analysis (ABA) (Wang et al. 2024). Verbal individuals on the autism spectrum and neurodiverse individuals endorse these types of naturalistic supports that consider variables such as the child's preference and that provide natural rewards (Schuck et al. 2022). Including motivational variables in support programs reduces avoidance and escape behaviors while simultaneously improving responsiveness.

Case Example: Emilio

Emilio was in kindergarten and greatly enjoyed buses. During free time and recess, he played alone, pretending that the bikes and other toys were buses. One day, he refused to share a bike with another student, stating that it was the end of the recess period, so the teacher punished Emilio by telling him that he could not talk about buses for the rest of the week. Instead of prohibiting this preferred activity, buses should have been embraced for use in teaching turn-taking and other academic subjects. Punishing and prohibiting this behavior resulted in morning school refusal and discontent at school. Furthermore, given Emilio's fascination with buses, prohibiting engagement in this activity required repeated verbal reprimands throughout the day. Clearly, his motivation was not considered, which caused further issues.

We began using this restricted interest to teach turn-taking (each child got a turn to give the driver a ticket, find a seat, and so on) and social conversation (asking peers if they took the bus, what bus passed their apartment, what type of transportation was their favorite, and so on). Following this change, which incorporated his restricted interest into socially appropriate activities, Emilio began to engage frequently with other students and, given his competence in the area, became a valued play partner.

Case Example: Sebastian

Sebastian was an autistic third grader who had not learned to read despite many attempts with commercial reading programs. His mother decided to take a different approach and used PRT to teach him to read during his favorite activity, cooking. She began by writing single words of ingredients while teaching him to sight-read the words. Sebastian quickly learned to read these words. Gradually, his mother added words to some of the items, such as "add pepperoni," "pour sauce," and "sprinkle cheese." After just a few months using the PRT motivational components of choice, natural rewards, interspersal, and rewarding attempts, Sebastian learned to decode, and his comprehension was able to be assessed by observing the completion of each direction.

Case Example: Brody

Brody was a middle schooler who spent his lunch recess pacing the perimeter of the playground. He reported to his psychiatrist that he "hated school" and would "rather die than go to school." Despite repeated parental requests to help him make friends, the school stated that he needed "time to decompress" during breaks. The psychiatrist encouraged the school to create a club around his restricted interest of coding, but that never came to fruition. Although the special education staff could not find a willing teacher to start a coding club, an aide volunteered to start a chess club. Brody took to this and quickly learned the rules, strategies, and winning moves. He began to comment, ask questions, and eventually teach the rules to other students. After beginning to engage in chess, he no longer spent his lunch periods alone but instead began to socialize with other students, including during class activities. School became enjoyable for him; he reported excitement about going to school and engaging with his peers and began meeting up with friends on weekends.

Incorporation of motivational components can explicitly be added to the individualized education program (IEP) or home program goals. The following are some considerations for goal development.

Support Programs

Support programs, whether they are a school IEP or an in-home program, must have the following characteristics.

Be Challenging

Too many programs include only maintenance activities or benchmarks that are too small for making any significant progress. Although PRT incorporates maintenance tasks, if everything is maintenance, the child will not progress.

Case Example: Wen

> Four-year-old Wen's verbal communication was delayed, and he demonstrated frequent echolalia, particularly when he did not understand a question. His parents prompted him to use verbal words frequently at home, and he used more than 50 spontaneously. When they did not understand what he wanted, such as when he said "car," they used an application on their phone that offered images they could use for specificity. With the pictures, Wen could clarify whether he wanted to go in the car to a fast-food restaurant, the park, or another location. This system worked well for him at home. At school, however, he was prompted to use his computerized augmentative and alternate communication (AAC) device to express his needs, even though his IEP required that he use verbal spoken communication in combination with the AAC device. Although he spent 6 hours per day in school, he was never prompted to use any verbal communication. Because verbal spoken communication required more prompting than the AAC device, this important acquisition area was being neglected. Consequently, his communication was not being challenged at school.

Include Socialization

Even though autism is characterized by social communication challenges, many children do not have social or social communication goals. School settings, with a plethora of peers, are an ideal place for teaching socialization, and the fact that verbal individuals on the spectrum almost universally report a desire for friends and social relationships underscores the importance of social support programs. Peer-mediated interventions, after-school programs, summer camps (Brookman et al. 2003; L.K. Koegel et al. 2012, 2019), clubs (Ashbaugh et al. 2017), home time with siblings (Baker et al. 1998), and any other social settings with similarly aged peers are ideal for teaching, prompting, and encouraging socialization and may be imperative for ensuring that social gains in clinic settings are used in everyday situations.

Case Example: Elijah

> Elijah attended middle school, and during observations we noted that he was regularly bullied by peers, even as he sat alone eating lunch. He complained that he wanted friends but did not know how to achieve this. The school responded that he needed "down time" at lunch, and they therefore were unwilling to start a program. However, they supported our request to help his social engagement by 1) reaching out to the students in one particular class (English) where he reported high levels of bullying and 2) creating a club for cartoon drawing, a strong talent of Elijah's. Elijah chose not to attend the presentation in his English class, but he and his parents gave us permission to discuss Elijah and his autism spectrum disorder (ASD). Right after the presentation in English, two students approached us and confided that they had no idea Elijah was on the autism spectrum, and they felt ashamed that they had been a part of the bullying. The day after the presentation, Elijah reported that his classmates were kind and supportive— a drastic change. Simultaneously, the cartoon drawing club that was held twice a week during lunch period became a popular club, and Elijah, with his giftedness in drawing, was the star member, idolized by the other members.

Be Practical

It is important to ensure that goals are practical and functional in the long run. Too many students reach adulthood without having the social communication or adaptive behaviors necessary to secure employment and live independently.

Case Example: Dean

> Dean was minimally verbal. His mother worked nights and complained that packing his lunch each day was exhausting and one of her least favorite chores. To support his mother and provide Dean with a lifelong skill, we used pictures to support him in the self-management activity of preparing and packing his own lunch. Using pictures that he turned over following each step, he was taught to independently prepare and pack a healthy lunch each evening and to clean up afterward. Aside from greatly helping his mother, which thrilled her, Dean learned a skill that would assist him in improving his independence.

Be Coordinated

Children learn much faster when everyone is on the same page. This means implementing the same goals across settings using the same techniques. This may seem like a small issue, but many children fall behind because one setting is different from another. For example, if nonverbal communication is rewarded in one setting and spoken communication in another, spoken communication may develop slowly. Similarly, if diapers are used in one setting and a child is expected to use the toilet in another, success may be slow or nonexistent. Keeping everyone on the same page is vital for accelerating the learning curve.

Case Example: Levi

> Levi's parents divorced when he was in preschool. His parents shared custody but had completely different values regarding raising children. Mom was quite "hands-off" and provided few opportunities for Levi to use communication. She did not follow through with programs for encouraging independent toileting and sleeping through the night. In fact, he wore a diaper at his mother's home, and she walked him in his stroller when he woke up during the night. At his father's home, Levi was encouraged to use verbal communication often and regularly throughout the day, was taken to the toilet on a schedule throughout the day, and was gently encouraged to go back to sleep when he awoke. Although some children can learn to engage in different routines in different settings, every transition caused a problem for Levi at his father's home because the expectations were different. After a day or two, he began using verbal, spoken communication at his father's home, successfully used the toilet, and slept through the night. Unfortunately, his gains were slow because of the inconsistencies across homes.

Parent Stress

Parent stress and low family well-being are common among parents of autistic children (MacKenzie and Eack 2022). Challenges for parents include management of challenging behaviors, financial burdens, loss of social contacts, decreased socialization, difficulties navigating the care system, and complications securing support services (MacKenzie and Eack 2022). Given the need for parents to actively participate in the teaching process, optimal outcomes depend on adequate mental health in order to implement and navigate a complex condition and system that changes over time. Research has fallen short of relieving parents of these psychological challenges thus far; however, several studies have implemented interventions that have led to some improvements in parental mental and physical health (Minjarez et al. 2013). For example, parent education that focuses on teaching parents how to effectively implement goals and manage behavior can be helpful for reducing day-to-day stress. Whereas requiring families to designate specific time periods for working with their child can increase stress, teaching families to provide opportunities on an ongoing basis in everyday situations and routines can decrease stress (R.L. Koegel et al. 1996). Other programs, such as mindfulness, parent support groups, social support, and matching parents for support or mentorship, can also can be helpful. Training extended families to provide emotional and child support can also be beneficial. Many families find respite to be useful, but it is important to find trained childcare providers so that parents are confident their child will be cared for properly when they are not there.

Fortunately, many siblings of children with disabilities enter the field of autism or disabilities and can personally relate to their patients. In the passage that follows, Dr. Ed Cook provides insight as a family member regarding the challenges families face, particularly when programs are offered that are not evidence-based.

Reflections on Services for Persons With Neurodevelopmental Disorders After Six Decades as a Brother, Psychiatrist, and Scientist, by Edwin H. Cook, M.D., and Niki P. Sabetfakhri, M.D., Ph.D.

My brother was born in 1961. That year, Solnit and Stark (1961) wrote about emotional responses to the birth of the "defective child" as a reason why physicians routinely recommended institutionalizing those with intellectual disability (ID) at the time of diagnosis during the first or second year of life. Our family fought strongly against such recommendations. I was 6 years old at the time and would not have occasion to cite this important paper until I wrote a case report in 1993 on the contribution of countertransference related to a "curative" treatment for autism, daily life therapy, and its role in the abuse of one of my patients (Cook et al. 1993).

The experience of my patient, and my written response to it, drew from my family's involvement in an earlier "cure" for neurodevelopmental disorders—the Doman-Delacato treatment—used for my brother's ID in the late 1960s. I recently came across a statement by many professional organizations warning about the Doman-Delacato treatment (Doman 1968). As I reflect on the statement now, there are several points that I wish had been disseminated to our family at the time, such as "promotional methods appear to put parents in a position where they cannot refuse such treatment without calling into question their adequacy and motivation as parents." To add to this point, there is an undeniable and profound sense of relief that accompanies being in a group of similar parents and hearing that others share your reasonable wishes for your child's (or sibling's) development to not be severely impaired. The impact of relieving this distress is something that I vividly recall, even decades later.

Another point that struck me in retrospect was: "It is asserted that if the therapy is not carried out as rigidly as prescribed, the child's potential will be damaged, and that anything less than 100% effort is useless." One of my strong recollections was of my mother being told that the treatment's failure to substantially improve my brother's cognition and language development was because of my family's failure to adhere to the program. However, we were strictly adherent to all the treatment guidelines. I am certain that this false blame contributed to a depressive episode for my mother. Knowledge of this professional warning back in 1968, before entry into the program, would have been very beneficial. However, by the time we encountered studies a few years later questioning the treatment's efficacy, we had too much emotional investment in the treatment and considered such studies to be an affront to something we "had" to believe in. Unfortunately, the issue of treatments overpromising results persists in the field of neurodevelopmental disorders.

My family and I always accepted my brother. Attempts to improve his development were primarily related to his safety. For example, his lack of pain sensitivity led to multiple cuts from the sharp edges of a can lid, necessitating constant supervision to prevent this and other such accidents. In his earliest years, frequent seizures called for the use of a helmet and a padded patio. Later, generalized seizures demanded our constant vigilance.

As a teenager, I devoted myself to developing better treatments for my brother, which ultimately led to my training as a psychiatrist and researcher. I observed that my brother became anxious with interruptions in his environment or routine, which stood in stark contrast to the repetitive behaviors he enjoyed. These observations, among others, inspired me to focus my clinical career on reducing emotional distress in individuals with ASD and comorbid ID. In the pursuit of better understanding and helping with rigidity and repetitive behaviors, I have treated and reported on the treatment of many patients with ASD and comorbid OCD using selective serotonin reuptake inhibitors (SSRIs) since their introduction in 1988. Unfortunately, my brother, who had comorbid epilepsy, experienced a sudden unexpected death in epilepsy (SUDEP) in 1989, prior to the possibility of an SSRI trial. Since then, my research career has been dedicated to better understanding the pathophysiology of ASD and its associated comorbidities, including the role of serotonin in neurodevelopmental disorders.

With the advancement of molecular genetic technology, many patients I have followed for decades now have ASD with or without ID that is associated with a specific de novo genetic variant. Although my brother died without a stored DNA sample, it is not completely by chance that I became involved in the dup15q Alliance, given that many with duplication of the 15q11-q13 region of maternal origin have a clinical presentation that overlaps with my brother's symptoms, including risk for SUDEP. It is my expectation that younger collaborators will move the field from identifying hundreds of specific genetic variants associated with ASD and ID to developing improved pharmacological treatments, particularly for the comorbid psychiatric symptoms that so often afflict those with developmental disorders. Additionally, I am hopeful that there will be improvements in access to optimal educational, behavioral (including better application of exposure therapy for those with anxiety disorders such as OCD), residential, vocational, and recreational supports. Although much work remains to be done to improve access to services throughout the lifespan, it is important to recognize that my brother and many others did not have access to public education until the landmark passage of PL 94-142 in 1975.

Marriages

The literature suggests that the parents of children with autism have higher rates of divorce, at rates that are almost twice those of parents of children without autism. Although divorce is most common among parents of neurotypical children early in the child's life, it continues through adulthood among parents of autistic children (Hartley et al. 2010). However, studies also show that parents who stay together and learn how to adapt to new and ongoing stresses and responsibilities may have higher levels of marital satisfaction (Saini et al. 2015), have stronger bonds, worry less about small things, and feel greater sensitivity and acceptance. Factors that may strengthen a relationship between parents of children with ASD include benefit finding (finding the positive in challenging events), social-emotional support (Ekas et al. 2015), and dyadic coping (Brown et al. 2020). Emphasizing resilience and actively assisting families in securing services, decreasing stress, improving confidence, learning procedures to manage their autistic child's behaviors, and establishing family support are important. Courses that teach effective communication, working together as a team, optimism and humor, support for each other, and developing family goals can be valuable in promoting resilience (Raffaele Mendez et al. 2019). High levels of child behavior problems are associated with lower levels of marital satisfaction (AlHorany et al. 2013; Sikora et al. 2013); thus, teaching parents to effectively implement procedures to reduce these behaviors is critical. In addition, marital satisfaction is correlated with low levels of stress and depression, so psychiatrists and other care providers can be instrumental in supporting families in seeking out services. However, these programs must be individualized to meet the family's needs and adapted for their personal situation and cultural values.

Cultural Issues

Another issue that has long been discussed is ensuring that intervention is adapted to meet a family's unique cultural norms and values. In the passage that follows, Dr. Dimitris Dimitriou addresses the importance of considering cultural issues during PRT training.

Cultural Issues, by Dimitris Dimitriou, M.D., Ph.D., Neurodevelopmental Pediatrician, President of the Cyprus Developmental and Behavioral Pediatrics Society, Yale University International Fellow, PRT International Program Coordinator

Increasing global autism awareness in recent years has also underlined the lack of services and expertise in many low- and middle-income countries around the world (Wallace et al. 2012). Especially in developing countries, appropriate training is needed in evidence-based practices (EBPs). Less than 10% of the world's population has access to EBPs such as PRT or ABA, and as autism becomes more visible, people face all sorts of cultural myths that may deter families from receiving a diagnosis and proper help. The cultural perspective shapes how parents may choose interventions and services and their cultural expectations of behavior. When trying to implement EBPs and train parents and professionals in using them, we face cultural and linguistic challenges for which there is limited research because most methods were developed in Western countries and are usually directed at an English-speaking population and a European American population (Davenport et al. 2018).

More research is imperative because there is an increase in culturally and linguistically diverse children in the United States as well. As we trained therapists and parents around the globe, it became clear that a multicultural approach to training was needed (Wilder et al. 2004) that would allow for PRT to be accordingly adapted, culturally and linguistically, while retaining its core components. This should be applied on two distinct levels: the training of parents and professionals and the implementation with children.

From personal experience, as a Greek-Cypriot neurodevelopmental pediatrician trained in the United States, I was faced with these exact issues upon my initial return to Greece and Cyprus in 2009. PRT was unknown in Greece and Cyprus, and only a handful of professionals were adequately trained at the time in EBPs. Families were struggling financially, and there was little family or community involvement. I tried to understand why, and the language barrier for the training was one of the key issues because most of the trainings had to be in English. This changed when we started using native speakers as trainers. That is, participants who understood the culture and nuances of the language could build better relationships not only with their child's therapists but also with the trainer. In addition, the cost of training at the time was quite high by local standards. The lack of standardized tests and the stigma associated with accessing therapy and with the diagnosis of ASD overall were also critical in delaying the therapy. More interestingly, most of the EBPs available at the time were considered not culturally appropriate, so parents and professionals alike found it difficult to follow and apply them. In fact, they usually believed that the methods were only appropriate for countries such as the United States.

In what some might consider a personal quest, I was trained in PRT and proceeded, under the guidance of Drs. Robert and Lynn Koegel, to help train others, initially in Greece and Cyprus and then in other countries all over the world, including the Middle East. The more I trained in PRT, the more I realized that it was extremely versatile in adapting to any cultural environment and began to see how it could be adapted linguistically.

We first had to consider certain factors that should always be investigated before beginning PRT. Because PRT is a naturalistic and evidence-based method that also directly involves the family and the community, many issues, as identified by researchers such as Saraceno et al. (2007), had to be addressed. These included, for example, parents' insufficient financial resources. PRT could multiply the hours of intervention a child received in a more generalized, culturally appropriate, and diverse setting while at the same time cutting the costs of lengthy sessions. This was especially important for families with limited resources. Parents were empowered, and children received more therapy hours. As one mother told me once: "Now we know what to do and how to do it."

Other issues included the need for appropriate professional training and the involvement of the community. PRT is a parent-mediated intervention that is proving to be more culturally sensitive and increasingly preferred by parents because the cultural values of the method align more easily with those of the families (R.L. Koegel et al. 1982). When we trained interdependent communities such as those in Cyprus, Greece, and Turkey, which still retain tight social group norms, the community became more helpful and understanding, rather than viewing autism as a stigma, and understood that an individual with autism is as important as anyone in the community (Papadopoulos et al. 2013). This proved to be particularly important because PRT endorses family and community involvement as well as autonomy, thus incorporating values from both more individualistic societies such as Anglo-American culture and more collective societies such as the Mediterranean, Middle Eastern, and Asian cultures, thereby rendering a more global treatment plan. This also led to a rapid spread of PRT in Greece, especially because of the community network that circulated the positive PRT results. In this way, PRT functioned to raise awareness because it lifted the stigma associated with autism treatment and helped it to be perceived as more natural.

Understanding Cultures

PRT is a culturally responsive, evidence-based intervention. Because it is a naturalistic method, following culturally relevant behaviors is inherent to PRT; therefore, it was easier for families and local therapists to adhere to PRT principles. However, for these cultural elements to be incorporated, they always had to be identified beforehand. Understanding a family's cultural background sheds light on how they interpret autism and what they perceive as helpful. We never assume that an ethnic group is homogeneous, but, rather, for every case we try to find therapists from that individual's specific group to assist us or someone else who may better understand their culture and language (Wang and Casillas 2013).

We also had to identify cultural factors relevant to training professionals before implementing our intervention strategies with children. It was evident in various cases, for example, that taking off one's shoes before entering a home and leaving them outside or by the door may not be appropriate in Western countries but was a cultural norm in areas such as the Middle East. We had to know these issues in advance in order to include them in the in-home programming using the PRT principles. Other examples include how we would greet someone and the words we would use, which are considered social interactions and differ in various cultures. Direct eye contact, which in Western culture is desirable, is viewed in some cultures as disrespectful, and children are characterized as shy and respectful when they avert their gaze during our intervention sessions. Physical prompting is also an issue; it is widely used in

Mediterranean and Latin cultures, particularly with boys, which may increase learned helplessness (DuBay et al. 2018). Thus, decreasing excessive prompting is often an area that needs to be addressed.

The role of the parents and the therapist also varies across cultures. In the Mediterranean, parents were not initially included as part of the therapy, as I experienced in Greece. In other cultures, gender roles were different. Sometimes, the father was not part of the intervention because this may have been considered emasculating or might suggest he was not knowledgeable enough to help with the child. Many times, the father was portrayed as the authority, or the one who would/should scold the child if they were not behaving correctly. The same issue was evident in areas where female therapists were preferred because they were considered more caring and loving. When we introduced PRT to these cultures, it also started to change their expectations about the roles of the families, therapists, and community, and they all became more involved (Bernier et al. 2010).

Even eating was culturally defined and quite diverse across cultures. Some cultures use utensils, while others use only the hands or only the right hand because the left hand is used during toileting and thus considered to be "dirty." Food habits may vary, and some types of food, such as pork or veal, may be prohibited. The same applies to *when* people eat; for example, during some holidays people eat only after sundown. Therapists not only should be flexible but also should know how to instill flexibility in an intervention plan right from the start, if possible, especially when planning for autonomy and adaptive abilities. This is something that PRT can do very well when applied correctly because it allows for more flexibility and child choices, thus reducing disruptive behaviors. It follows not only the child but also the family.

Understanding culture and other factors, such as gender, religion, food, location, childrearing practices, ethnicity, language, community structure, and even weather, is extremely important because these factors influence the impact of autism on a family or the training. Culture also has an impact on what people expect of children and how people grieve, perceive the stigma and discrimination toward, and accept the ASD diagnosis (Matson et al. 2017). Some parents believe their child never had autism, despite the official diagnosis. Others believe it is an act of God or a punishment for something they have done. Once we know the roles that ethnicity and culture play in the autism stigma, these attitudes may be moderated, which may lead to more efficient intervention services, as well as to more willingness to access services (Kang-Yi et al. 2018).

When we train families and therapists in PRT, one thing is clear: we are there to listen to them. We are not there to judge their practices nor to change them but, rather, to use them for the child's benefit according to PRT principles. All this also proved significant in training culturally diverse children and professionals. When we explained what PRT could do for them, they felt more comfortable using it. It feels "right," as one parent said. PRT followed the family's schedule and tried to resolve obvious issues without going against parents' beliefs. This helped with parental and community denial because community members felt comfortable helping these families and began believing that children could improve. By using PRT, the community started changing its belief that nothing could be done. By better understanding what *could* be done, they became less judgmental and more accepting of parents of children with autism.

Language

Language, especially its structure, is a critical factor in this procedure. One of the first things we had to tackle when applying PRT was the language milestones, even though these are consistent across languages. Following commands and being "disciplined" was more important in some cultures than talking. In many cultures, it was acceptable for boys especially to be language delayed, and parents had to understand that language had to be reinforced at the same time as following commands and what was considered communication.

If the trainer is not a native speaker of the trainees' language, they need to be very well informed about how the language is pronounced and its structure because this may interfere with the child's training. For example, some languages, such as Greek or Turkish, may use longer words right from the start or may use different words than we use in English. In Turkish, the word for "I want" is *istiyorum*, and in Greek, it is *thelo*. Both words are difficult in comparison with their English equivalent. Also, in some languages, the use of pronouns may be obligatory, as in English, whereas in others, such as Greek and Turkish, it may not. This does not make the language more "difficult" to teach, but it does change the way it is presented to the child. For example, in PRT we model words the child should use, such as "I want." In Greek, it is only one word, "thelo," and the pronoun "I" is implied by the ending of the verb. Other languages, Russian, for example, may lack basic verbs such as "to be" or "to have"; thus, when you're saying, "I'm a doctor," the direct translation would be "I doctor." The verb "to be" is implied by the noun. The structure of a language may be quite different; Turkish, which is an agglutinating language, usually requires suffixes to be added at the ends of words. This becomes important in cases such as reinforcing attempts, which is a core component of PRT. A similar issue had to be resolved in cases of languages such as Greek, which have inclinations.

As a result, although the core components of the PRT method remain unaltered, the examples provided when training professionals should be drawn from research conducted before starting any training in a foreign country. Being aware of these differences, I turned to Dr. Lynn Koegel for help on how to teach PRT in other countries and cultures. Her answer regarding languages was clear: if we use the motivational component, there will be no problem. Find out what the child wants, she said, and that will guide you and the words you should use. What we search for, she added, is communication; the words will follow. The English language has a lot of single-phoneme words such as "talk" or "walk" that double as nouns and verbs. However, the Greek language has long words and may be considered rather difficult to teach, so I opted for more verbs, especially those that began with labial movements and were easier to copy, such as "pata," which means "click," or "papi," which means "duck." For Turkish, I used more abbreviated forms of verbs rather than the more formal ones. This gave the approach a versatility in generalizing words while following the PRT principles of modeling and motivation.

PRT involves the community and the families, and in countries that are culturally diverse, where the language spoken at home may be different from the language spoken at school, we ask the parents to provide us with the words they use in their daily lives. By being culturally responsive, naturalistic, and parent- and community-mediated, PRT increases participation and expectations among the families of children with autism as well as their communities. It is now available worldwide, with manuals and books translated into various languages, but most of all, it is an EBP that is adaptable to people's cultures and values with minimal effort.

Daily Life

Although the focus of this book is on PRT for teaching communication and academics and addressing interfering behaviors, sleep and eating issues also are common among individuals on the autism spectrum, and it is important for psychiatrists and others to discuss these with families. Challenges with eating and sleeping can greatly affect child development and behavior, as well as parental mental health (Guller and Yaylaci 2022), and should be addressed early on. Various behavioral programs are available that can assist with these issues. For example, a systematic review showed that parents can serve as intervention agents at home, using strategies that include sleep hygiene modifications (e.g., fading long bedtime routines and parental presence, gradual extinction, darkening the room, visual aids, positive behavioral support, developing a regular bedtime routine, relaxation, distraction, self-management) (Hunter et al. 2020).

Behavioral interventions have also been helpful, to various degrees, for feeding difficulties, which are sometimes caused by sensory issues.

Examples include video modeling with nonpreferred foods (e.g., a video of a child eating a nonpreferred food while making positive comments about it), reinforcement for trying or eating a nonpreferred food, fading in nonpreferred foods, systematic and gradual desensitization to new foods, and rewarding eating new foods with preferred foods, items, or activities (L.K. Koegel and LaZebnik 2023; R.L. Koegel et al. 2012; Williams and Seiverling 2023). However, feeding challenges are complicated, and a thorough understanding of the issues causing and maintaining them is essential.

Summary

Psychiatrists and other care providers can support parents and caregivers by recommending therapeutic day-to-day interactions that can make a difference in the long term. These should include culturally sensitive methods for managing behaviors, including reducing interfering behaviors, improving sleep and diet, and supporting academics and communication. Many of these interactions do not come naturally to parents because children on the autism spectrum tend to engage in fewer social interactions than their neurotypical peers, but they can be arranged in everyday situations. Ensuring that the PRT motivational procedures are being incorporated will result in faster learning and improved affect.

Another important issue relates to the stress experienced by parents and care providers of children on the autism spectrum. Parent and caregiver involvement in their child's program is highly beneficial, and psychiatrists and providers should recommend support for the entire family. Divorce is more common among the parents of autistic children than among parents of neurotypical children; however, the small amount of literature that has focused on parents who successfully stay married suggests that these couples have closer bonds with their partners and more appreciation, happiness, and fulfillment. Although it is difficult to entirely decrease the stress related to having a child with disabilities, psychiatrists can write strengths-based reports, make intervention recommendations, and suggest researched methods that improve parents' optimism. Within a marriage, increased happiness can be related to many factors, including equally dividing tasks, respecting and working together with one's partner, focusing on the positives of the child, having social support, and reducing other stressors such as financial concerns and other mental health conditions

(Saini et al. 2015). Psychiatrists and health care providers can make suggestions and support parents in understanding and actively addressing issues that are likely to improve their marital happiness. Education of the wider public is also needed to support and include individuals on the spectrum and their families (Curley et al. 2023; L.K. Koegel and LaZebnik 2023). As the incidence of ASD continues to rise, these needs are becoming even more pressing.

References

AlHorany AK, Hassan SA, Bataineh MZ: A review on factors affecting marital adjustment among parents of autistic children and gender effects. Life Sci J 10(1):400–405, 2013

Ashbaugh K, Koegel R, Koegel L: Increasing social integration for college students with autism spectrum disorder. Behav Dev Bull 22(1):183–196, 2017 28642808

Baker MJ, Koegel RL, Koegel LK: Increasing the social behavior of young children with autism using their obsessive behaviors. Journal of the Association for Persons With Severe Handicaps 23(4):300–308, 1998

Bernier R, Mao A, Yen J: Psychopathology, families, and culture: autism. Child Adolesc Psychiatr Clin N Am 19(4):855–867, 2010 21056350

Brookman L, Boettcher M, Klein E, et al: Facilitating social interactions in a community summer camp setting for children with autism. J Posit Behav Interv 5(4):249–252, 2003

Brown M. Whiting J, Kahumoku-Fessler E, et al: A dyadic model of stress, coping, and marital satisfaction among parents of children with autism. Fam Relat 69(1):138–150, 2020

Cook EH Jr, Kieffer JE, Charak DA, et al: Autistic disorder and post-traumatic stress disorder. J Am Acad Child Adolesc Psychiatry 32(6):1292–1294, 1993 8282677

Curley K, Colman R, Rushforth A, et al: Stress reduction interventions for parents of children with autism spectrum disorder: a focused literature review. Youth (Basel) 3(1):246–260, 2023

Davenport M, Mazurek M, Brown A, et al: A systematic review of cultural considerations and adaptation of social skills interventions for individuals with autism spectrum disorder. Res Autism Spectr Disord 52:23–33, 2018

Doman G: The Doman-Delacato treatment of neurologically handicapped children. Neurology 18(12):1214–1216, 1968 4236482

DuBay M, Watson LR, Zhang W: In search of culturally appropriate autism interventions: perspectives of Latino caregivers. J Autism Dev Disord 48(5):1623–1639, 2018 29188586

Ekas NV, Timmons L, Pruitt M, et al: The power of positivity: predictors of relationship satisfaction for parents of children with autism spectrum disorder. J Autism Dev Disord 45(7):1997–2007, 2015 25601217

Guller B, Yaylaci F: Eating and sleep problems, related factors, and effects on the mental health of the parents in children with autism spectrum disorder. Int J Dev Disabil 70(3):406–415, 2022 38699491

Hartley SL, Barker ET, Seltzer MM, et al: The relative risk and timing of divorce in families of children with an autism spectrum disorder. J Fam Psychol 24(4):449–457, 2010 20731491

Hunter JE, McLay LK, France KG, et al: Systematic review of the collateral effects of behavioral sleep interventions in children and adolescents with autism spectrum disorder. Res Autism Spectr Disord 79:101677, 2020

Kang-Yi CD, Grinker RR, Beidas R, et al: Influence of community-level cultural beliefs about autism on families' and professionals' care for children. Transcult Psychiatry 55(5):623–647, 2018 29972327

Koegel LK, LaZebnik C: Hidden Brilliance: Unlocking the Intelligence of Autism. New York, Harper Wave, 2023

Koegel LK, Vernon T, Koegel RL, et al: Improving social engagement and initiations between children with autism spectrum disorder and their peers in inclusive settings. J Posit Behav Interv 14(4):220–227, 2012 25328380

Koegel LK, Glugatch LB, Koegel RL, et al: Targeting IEP social goals for children with autism in an inclusive summer camp. J Autism Dev Disord 49(6):2426–2436, 2019 30927180

Koegel RL, Schreibman L, Britten KR, et al: A comparison of parent training to direct child treatment, in Educating and Understanding Autistic Children. San Diego, CA, College-Hill Press, 1982, pp 260–279

Koegel RL, Bimbela A, Schreibman L: Collateral effects of parent training on family interactions. J Autism Dev Disord 26(3):347–359, 1996 8792265

Koegel RL, Bharoocha AA, Ribnick CB, et al: Using individualized reinforcers and hierarchical exposure to increase food flexibility in children with autism spectrum disorders. J Autism Dev Disord 42(8):1574–1581, 2012 22042309

MacKenzie KT, Eack SM: Interventions to improve outcomes for parents of children with autism spectrum disorder: a meta-analysis. J Autism Dev Disord 52(7):2859–2883, 2022 34189683

Matson JL, Matheis M, Burns CO, et al: Examining cross-cultural differences in autism spectrum disorder: a multinational comparison from Greece, Italy, Japan, Poland, and the United States. Eur Psychiatry 42:70–76, 2017 28212508

Minjarez MB, Mercier EM, Williams SE, et al: Impact of pivotal response training group therapy on stress and empowerment in parents of children with autism. J Posit Behav Interv 15(2):71–78, 2013

Papadopoulos C, Foster J, Caldwell K: "Individualism-collectivism" as an explanatory device for mental illness stigma. Community Ment Health J 49(3):270–280, 2013 22837106

Raffaele Mendez LM, Berkman K, Lam GYH, et al: Fostering resilience among couples coparenting a young child with autism: an evaluation of Together We Are Stronger. Am J Fam Ther 47(3):165–182, 2019

Saini M, Stoddart KP, Gibson M, et al: Couple relationships among parents of children and adolescents with autism spectrum disorder: findings from a scoping review of the literature. Res Autism Spectr Disord 17:142–157, 2015

Saraceno B, van Ommeren M, Batniji R, et al: Barriers to improvement of mental health services in low-income and middle-income countries. Lancet 370(9593):1164–1174, 2007 17804061

Schuck RK, Tagavi DM, Baiden KMP, et al: Neurodiversity and autism intervention: reconciling perspectives through a naturalistic developmental behavioral intervention framework. J Autism Dev Disord 52(10):4625–4645, 2022 34643863

Sikora D, Moran E, Orlich F, et al: The relationship between family functioning and behavior problems in children with autism spectrum disorders. Res Autism Spectr Disord 7(2):307–315, 2013

Solnit A, Stark M: Mourning and the birth of a defective child. Psychoanal Study Child 16:523–537, 1961

U.S. Congress, Public Law 94-142, Education for All Handicapped Children Act (November 29, 1975). U.S. Congress, Senate, Education for All Handicapped Children Act S. 6, 94th Congress, 1st Session, June 2, 1975, Report No. 94-168.

Wallace S, Fein D, Rosanoff M, et al: A global public health strategy for autism spectrum disorders. Autism Res 5(3):211–217, 2012 22605577

Wang HT, Casillas N: Asian American parents' experiences of raising children with autism: multicultural family perspective. J Asian Afr Stud 48(5):594–606, 2013

Wang L, Li S, Wang C: Using pivotal response treatment to improve language functions of autistic children in special schools: a randomized controlled trial. J Autism Dev Disord 54(6):2081–2093, 2024 37101061

Wilder LK, Dyches TT, Obiakor FE, et al: Multicultural perspectives on teaching students with autism. Focus Autism Other Dev Disabl 19(2):105–113, 2004

Williams K, Seiverling L: Behavior analytic feeding interventions: current state of the literature. Behav Modif 47(4):983–1011, 2023 35674422

Index